YOUR HEART IS THE
SIZE OF YOUR FIST

MARTINA SCHOLTENS, MD

YOUR HEART
Is the Size of
YOUR FIST

*A Doctor Reflects on Ten Years
at a Refugee Clinic*

BRINDLE
& GLASS

Brindle & Glass
An imprint of TouchWood Editions
Brindleandglass.com

The information in this book is true and complete to the best of the author's knowledge. All recommendations are made without guarantee on the part of the author or the publisher.

Edited by Lynne Van Luven
Cover design by Tree Abraham
Cover image by Rebecca Wellman
Interior design by Pete Kohut
Proofread by Claire Philipson

Permission for the use of quote from Susan Cain's *Quiet: The Power of Introverts in a World That Can't Stop Talking* (New York: Crown Publishers, 2012) has been kindly granted by Penguin Random House LLC.

LIBRARY AND ARCHIVES CANADA CATALOGUING IN PUBLICATION
Scholtens, Martina, author
Your heart is the size of your fist : a doctor reflects on ten years at a refugee clinic / Martina Scholtens.

Issued in print and electronic formats.
ISBN 978-1-927366-68-4 (softcover).

1. Scholtens, Martina. 2. Refugees—Medical care—Canada—Anecdotes. 3. Clinics—Canada—Anecdotes 4. Physician and patient—Anecdotes. 5. Physicians—Canada—Biography. I. Title.

RA564.9.R43S74 2017   362.1086'914   C2017-903017-5

We acknowledge the financial support of the Government of Canada through the Canada Book Fund and the Canada Council for the Arts, and of the Province of British Columbia through the British Columbia Arts Council and the Book Publishing Tax Credit.

Canada Council for the Arts   Conseil des Arts du Canada   BRITISH COLUMBIA ARTS COUNCIL

The interior pages of this book have been printed on 100% post-consumer recycled paper, processed chlorine free, and printed with vegetable-based inks.

PRINTED IN CANADA

21 20 19 18 17   2 3 4 5

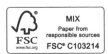

MIX
Paper from responsible sources
FSC® C103214

For Pete

PREFACE

I WORKED AS A FAMILY DOCTOR at Bridge Refugee Clinic in Vancouver, Canada, from 2005 to 2015. The clinic provides care to one to two thousand new refugees arriving in British Columbia each year. I started fresh out of residency, spent my thirties there, and ended up becoming the clinic's medical coordinator. As a clinical instructor with the Faculty of Medicine at the University of British Columbia, I supervised a steady stream of students and residents over the years. I heard and told a lot of stories.

My clinic days end with charting—updating the patients' medical records with their concerns, my findings, and our plan. But I often follow that with writing down for myself the details of something that moved me that day. Sometimes I write to reflect, sometimes to memorialize the patient.

There is a third reason I write: advocacy. I support refugees, the Canadians who welcome them, and a robust refugee policy. With increasing media coverage of refugees following cuts to federal health coverage in 2012, Canada's commitment to Syrian refugees in 2015, and policy changes south of the border in 2017, I read and listened to a myriad of opinions on our country's newest residents. Much of what I encountered was inconsistent with what I saw in my exam room. I thought my vantage point might be worth sharing.

This book was written with the utmost respect for patient privacy, for what the Hippocratic Oath calls "holy secrets." While all events and conversations depicted in this book occurred in some form during my decade at the clinic, details have been altered so that the patient cannot be identified. Some stories are a composite of multiple patient encounters, about an experience common to many refugees. Others stories are shared with patient permission; even then, I have not used their names. I have made every effort in the details included, withheld, and modified to preserve the trust of both the doctor-patient and the writer-reader relationship.

1

EAGER TO PRACTISE HIS ENGLISH, Yusef waived my offer of an Arabic interpreter for his appointment with me, as he usually did. After a year in Surrey, a suburb of Vancouver, Canada, he and his wife, Junah, had mastered the language enough to order lamb from Save On Meats and to ask the bus driver for directions to the refugee clinic at Main and Broadway in Vancouver. They did not, in fact, have the fluency for a doctor visit.

I ushered the couple into my exam room, where they sat down, beaming.

Yusef came straight to the point: "I want to kill you."

"Pardon me?"

"I want to kill you." He gazed straight at me. I stared back, wondering if I'd need to use the panic button hidden beneath my desk. He was composed and spoke quietly; it was hard to know whether to take this as reassuring or chilling.

"I try, this week," he went on. "Twice, I try to kill you." His wife nodded.

I thought back over my week. It had been uneventful. "Tell me more."

He pointed to the phone. "I try to kill you. But no one answer."

"Oh! Call me! You tried to call me!"

"Yes, yes, call," he corrected himself. "What mean kill?"

"Murder. Make me dead."

They laughed until they had to dab at their eyes with tissues.

I laughed too, a chuckle of relief. I marvelled that they were crying with laughter at a joke about death. A year ago, I'd never have believed it.

"YUSEF HADDAD?" I CALLED INTO the waiting room after consulting my day sheet. "Junah Haddad?"

The clinic waiting room was furnished with salvaged church pews, the oak worn smooth from years of waiting on God and the doctor. The furniture had struck me as incongruous when I started at the clinic, but I'd since decided it wasn't that unnatural a fit. Church and clinic were both places where people gathered to seek answers, sites of congregation and confession.

A family of four sat patiently on the pew at the far end of the waiting room, facing me, beneath a window overlooking the parking lot. They didn't seem bothered that the clinic was running fifteen minutes late. They looked resigned, like they were accustomed to waiting. They fit the demographic of the new family scheduled to see me that afternoon: an Arabic couple in their forties, with two teenage children. They stood uncertainly as I repeated their names. They looked tired and bewildered.

They'd arrived in Canada earlier in the week and were staying at Welcome House, transitional housing in downtown Vancouver, until they found permanent housing. I knew their past few days would have been a confusing rush of orientation sessions and registration for everything from a bank account to health insurance. The husband held a transparent sleeve containing the paperwork the family had been issued in the past week.

I extended my hand and introduced myself. "I'm Dr. Scholtens." Sometimes Muslim men refused my offered hand, believing that Islam forbids non-essential contact with a woman who is not wife or family. Yusef didn't hesitate to grasp it. He didn't smile, but his eyes met mine. He was tall, over six feet, with wide shoulders and a narrow waist. He was well-groomed, hair slicked back, dark moustache neatly trimmed. He wore a button-down shirt and navy trousers. His shoes gleamed with fresh polish.

Junah's handshake was quick and tentative. A white head-scarf with a green print band was wrapped tightly around her face, without a wisp of hair showing. She was almost certainly a brunette, but with her blue eyes and fair skin, I could imagine her as a blonde.

The teenage son was almost as tall as his dad, but his face was boyish and he stood awkwardly. His younger sister, in jeans and a pink headscarf, studied me with interest. I smiled at them.

"And this is Hani, the interpreter," I said. Hani, a young Somali woman, stepped forward and spoke in Arabic. She'd started at our clinic as a patient four years ago, but as her English was excellent and she couldn't work as a dentist until she'd satisfied the Canadian professional requirements, she'd returned as an interpreter. We'd worked together for two years.

"Let's start the visit with the whole family," I proposed, "and then I can see you individually for specific issues as needed." All four Haddads followed me to my exam room.

My assigned room was one of a dozen in the Raven Song Community Health Centre. It was in the rear of the building, positioned between the men's washroom and the exit. This had always struck me as vaguely symbolic of the marginalization of my patients, and of the odd orbit of my medical career, on the fringe of regular family medicine.

I only saw newly arrived refugees. I was one of five physicians in British Columbia who did this work. We all practiced at Bridge Clinic, housed in the southeast corner of the Raven Song building. We all worked part-time because the work was difficult. I saw patients three days a week and stayed home with my kids the other four.

The clinic saw approximately 1,800 new patients a year who came from around the world, mostly from United Nations refugee camps. It was a few blocks from Vancouver General Hospital, in the heart of the city. The specialists to whom I referred patients were stacked a dozen layers high in the medical office buildings just down Broadway. At noon I could strike out in any direction and find a satisfying lunch in minutes: congee, bagels, sushi, ramen. The neighbourhoods held heritage homes with porches and wildflower gardens set in a vibrant hub of traffic and sirens.

Exam room 146 was unassuming. It was smaller than the washroom across the hall and designed by someone who had never interacted with patients. A sink, cupboards, and a computer desk took up the far wall. The paper towel dispenser had been installed with an inch to spare above the counter, so that a paper jam had to be awkwardly dislodged after every crank of the handle. A plum-coloured vinyl exam table hugged the left wall, with two chairs wedged between the foot of the table and the sink. Whenever I did a Pap test, I had to reconfigure the room in order to extend the stirrups. The sharps container was mounted on the wall above the pair of chairs, precisely located so that seated adults struck their heads whenever they shifted position. Two more chairs were pushed against the opposite wall.

A red Tupperware box on the shelf held my preferred stationery, next to a Richard Scarry picture book for pediatric patients. At one point I had bought an aquarium, a self-sustaining ecosystem developed by NASA where shrimp, algae, and bacteria lived symbiotically in a sealed glass globe; I thought it would be a peaceful and harmonious point in the room. The shrimp kept dying, though, and this seemed an ominous message in a doctor's office, so now my counter held only the usual tray of cotton swabs and rubber tourniquets. The respiratory therapist who used the room on my off days had hung educational posters on the walls. My colleague had grumbled at these when he poked his head in that morning: "Some of our patients have seen lungs, you know. Those pictures could trigger flashbacks."

Yusef and Junah took the chairs beneath the sharps container, their daughter sat under the emphysema poster, and the son hauled himself onto the exam table. I took the chair at the computer desk, Hani next to me, and pulled up the family's file.

The clinic nurses visit Welcome House to screen new arrivals shortly after their arrival in Canada, before their first appointment with a physician. I looked over their note. It began with the standard checklist:

Country of origin: Iraq
Country of transit: Egypt
Date of arrival in Canada: September 23
Occupation: Husband - journalist. Wife - engineer.
Children: Nadia (14), Layth (16) - developmental delay?
Trauma? ✔

It went on to outline the medical history of each family member: surgeries, medication, chronic disease, allergies. My tasks today would be to determine whether further testing needed to be added to the routine screening blood work, renew any prescriptions, address any urgent issues, and outline a plan for future care.

Yusef and Junah deflected my questions about their medical histories. Their only concern was for their son, Layth.

"He can't learn," Hani interpreted. "Never went to school."

Layth sat on the edge of the exam table, grinning, legs dangling. He was as sturdy as a man, charming as a boy. I observed him as his parents described his childhood: late to walk, late to talk, odd behaviour, such as hand flapping. He had no formal medical diagnosis. He had been inadmissible for school in their Iraqi hometown of Mosul. Junah had put her engineering career on hold to care for him. His widely spaced eyes, short neck, and monobrow made me wonder whether he had a genetic condition.

"Do any of your relatives have similar problems?" They didn't.

"Were you related to each other before you were married?" Approximately 30 percent of marriages in Iraq are between first cousins. Consanguinity—literally "common blood"—was not unusual among my patients, especially those from Middle Eastern, West Asian, and North African cultures with a long-standing tradition of marriage between blood relatives.

"Their mothers are sisters," confirmed Hani.

I arranged for Layth to return to see me for a full assessment. I expected he'd need referrals to Pediatrics and Medical Genetics.

"Their settlement worker told them he will go to school, but they don't believe that is possible," said Hani.

"Yes, he will go to school," I confirmed. "In Canada, every child has a right to education. They'll make accommodations for him—an aide, or special classes."

After Hani relayed this, the parents turned to me with tears in their eyes. "Thank you, Doctor," said Yusef, bowing his head and shoulders toward me.

"Thank you," echoed Junah softly, also in English.

I knew I didn't deserve any personal thanks. I was just lucky enough to be a frontline representative of the country that had offered them refuge; I was one of the first faces of hospitality newcomers met when they arrived.

I printed off the lab requisitions and tapped my notes into the computer. "Is this the whole family?" I asked, as the visit wound down. "Is anyone missing?" I'd learned not to assume that the family in front of me was intact. Older children sometimes remained in their home country to complete university. Sometimes an infant born after the family registered with the United Nations had to be left behind because the parents didn't know they had to complete additional paperwork. Many patients had lived communally with extended family, but their elderly parents were too frail to travel or unwilling to leave their home.

Hani repeated my question in Arabic, and the entire family began to weep. It was a chorus: sobbing from Nadia, unrestrained bawling from Layth, low moaning from Junah, rapid speech from Yusuf as tears ran down his face. I sensed there was relief in the crying, as if they'd been waiting for an invitation to spill over.

During the exchange of Arabic, I waited. Crying no longer alarmed me. Some days every patient cried. The box of tissues on my counter got as much play as my stethoscope.

The story was this: Sami Haddad had been buried before his twelfth birthday.

Yusef had been a journalist in Mosul, in northern Iraq, for almost twenty years. He'd covered the culture and politics beats for *Nineveh Radio*. Yusef was not the first Iraqi journalist I'd seen at the refugee clinic. I knew that just being associated with an Iraqi newspaper or TV station that was seen by anti-government forces as supportive of the US-backed Iraqi government was risky. According to the Committee to Protect Journalists, 102 Iraqi journalists had been murdered over the past decade.[1]

A year and a half ago, as Yusef and his eleven-year-old son, Sami, played soccer in the courtyard of their home after dinner, a car pulled up. Masked gunmen dragged Yusef and Sami into the vehicle. They were held for three days, beaten, and dumped on the bank of the Tigris River. Sami died of a head injury. When Yusef had recovered from his injuries enough to travel, he fled to Egypt with his family. They registered with the United Nations Refugee Agency and arrived in Canada eighteen months later.

I knew that Yusef had heavily abbreviated the story, not for my benefit but to spare his wife and children. I didn't press for details; I knew that eventually he would release them to me for safekeeping.

I'd listened to terrible stories, one after another, for years. The horror of this story, though, was magnified by Biblical themes: the Tigris River of the Garden of Eden; Nineveh of Jonah and the whale; violence on an Old Testament scale. It almost felt mythical. But the father in front of me opened his wallet, extracted a snapshot from the billfold compartment, and passed it to me

The boy in the picture was climbing a date palm: flip-flops, lean legs, long shorts, a yellow T-shirt. His head was silhouetted against the sky, hair a mess of black waves.

"That week he die," Yusef said. "Last photo."

As a physician, I kept my personal life strictly separate from work. I didn't wear my wedding band, and there were no family portraits on my desk. I had children too, though—three of them at the time. My greatest fear was that I'd be unable to protect them from harm.

There was nothing I could say or do to make his son's death right. "I'm so sorry," I said. Ingrained professionalism kept my voice steady; they were only three words, but I looked at Yusef as I said them. I could see that they were enough.

That night, I ate dinner with my family at the beach near our home in Deep Cove, a thirty-minute commute from the clinic. After we'd cleared the picnic table, my husband, Pete, and I walked out to the dock and watched our kids playing along the shore. Our six-year-old son found a cluster of dandelions gone to seed; he hunched over, snapping the hollow milky stems and double fisting his prize.

"I'm going to make a wish!" said Leif. "I wish for . . ." I could see him searching for something extravagant. "A chocolate cake!" He puffed energetically, spit flying, and his lips almost touching the white fluff.

"Look, a school of wishes!" He watched them drift off in a hazy clump. "Hey! The wishes are all hugging each other!" And then he spotted some goslings and trotted off down the beach.

How wonderful to wish for chocolate cake, to have to think hard for something to wish for, to have all your needs met, to have no cares or sickness or worries to wish away. My children and their unspoiled interactions with the world were the most potent antidote to the suffering I witnessed at work and sometimes carried home with me like a bloodstain on my sleeve.

But once the kids were put to bed, and I settled on the couch to watch Netflix, I clicked past all the romantic comedies and TV sitcoms. I deliberated between *Blood Diamond, Lost Boys of Sudan*, and a Holocaust documentary. The awfulness overwhelmed me, but it felt disrespectful to enjoy something light after the day's work, and I gravitated toward the heavy fare out of a sense of obligation. I knew it wasn't good for me, but out of a perverse sense of solidarity with my patients, I immersed myself in scenes of injustice until bedtime.

2

HAD A SECRET: I WASN'T working at the clinic because I *had a heart for* refugees.

When people learned what field I worked in, they often assumed that I did and commended me for it with an admiration that made me uncomfortable. It was too awkward to protest what was meant to be a compliment, so I let it go. Having *a heart for refugees* suggests that one is blessed with divine direction, certainty, and servitude—none of which I felt I could honestly own up to. My career has been a guided drift. While in hindsight there appears to be a logical development to my career path, as I've moved along it I've never been able to see beyond the next six weeks. Refugee medicine was never a goal I set my sights on. Yet here I was, with a job I loved so much that my six-year-old asked me, "I can never remember. Do they pay you to go to work, or do you pay them to let you work?"

People love the narrative of a child being called to the medical profession. "Did you always know that you wanted to be a doctor?" I'm asked regularly. In fact, I didn't consider medicine until I was twenty-one.

I grew up in a conservative religious community in the Fraser Valley. I graduated from high school in a class of forty; every one of us was white and Dutch Canadian. Most of my classmates were engaged by twenty-one, with three or four kids by our ten-year reunion. As time went on, I would lag further and further behind those peers.

I understood from kindergarten that if I were to pursue a career, the options were limited to those traditionally dominated by women, such as teaching elementary school or nursing. Once I married, I was expected to leave my career for motherhood. I didn't protest this as a child; virtually all women in my community were homemakers. And I didn't know anyone—man or woman—in medicine.

I always had an inkling, though, that my path wouldn't be traditional. First of all, my father was a university professor. Even when I was in elementary school, the potential track of education appeared infinite to me, extending far past high school.

"Could I speak to Dr. Byl, please?" his students would say when I answered the phone in the evening.

"He's a teacher, not a doctor," I'd say. "But you can speak to him."

I loved learning. I could remember where I sat and what I wore in Grade 8 science when Mr. Mans explained why a sugar cube dissolved more quickly in hot water than in cold. The concept of sugar crystals being bombarded by water molecules whose velocity increased with temperature gave me joy, although I was socially aware enough to keep it to myself.

In high school, there were only five of us in Physics 12. We all had a literal front row seat to Mr. Koat, who taught with pleasure and marked with precision, down to the quarter point. At lunch one day my friends and I discovered a large empty barrel in the school parking lot. I climbed inside and they rolled me across the playing field. Mr. Koat was on lunch monitor duty and hurried over as I emerged from the barrel.

"Martina, I saw what you did there," he said. "With your aptitude for science and sense of adventure, perhaps you should consider becoming an astronaut."

I laughed, but he didn't. Someone thought astronautics a viable career option for me. I was astonished. The narrow set of possibilities I'd grown up with started to fan open.

For an English 12 assignment, we were to write an essay on a book that had influenced us. I wrote that I had been scarred by the fairy tale *Cinderella*, that I'd identified with the wicked stepsisters rather than the beautiful, meek heroine. When Mr. Schön handed back our essays, next to my score was a comment, circled emphatically: "Worthy of publication."

Again, I was presented with a possibility I'd never entertained. I submitted it to the *Vancouver Sun*, and they published it. This led to my first two reader responses, handwritten letters forwarded by the *Sun*: one from an elderly woman who called me a spoiled brat, and the other from a man who said he could relate to my experience and suggested we meet. (We didn't.)

I was lucky enough to have teachers who championed their

students, who recognized what I enjoyed and excelled at, and suggested how that might be expanded.

In high school, I had no clear idea about my future career, and that didn't bother me. I loved learning and I simply planned to pursue higher education for as long as possible. Being equipped for a career would be a byproduct of my education, not the goal of it. But which direction to go? Arts or science?

Lying on the floor of my bedroom in Grade 12, flipping through university catalogues, everything appealed to me: English, chemistry, business. It was my first step into that funnel of adulthood, where the act of choosing one thing went hand-in-hand with rejecting others. I thought I had to commit exclusively to one discipline—career monogamy—and I was sorry to have to break up with other subjects that I loved.

I decided to major in English. My freshman year at university was saturated with the arts. I studied *Silas Marner*, took a drawing class on Tuesday nights, and played Mote in the production of *A Midsummer Night's Dream*, in which I sang and flitted across the stage in a swimsuit and gauzy wings. One day that spring, I walked into my English classroom just after it had been vacated by a chemistry class. On the board an elaborate equation was worked out, rows and rows of characters, and at the bottom, after the equals sign, was the singular, right answer.

At that moment, I realized how much I longed for right answers, how much the softness and imprecision of the arts frustrated me. I had a vague sense of pursuing the "real thing"; I couldn't articulate what it was, but I recognized it when I brushed by it. It would take me years to realize that the truest answers do lie in the arts. When I registered for the next semester that spring, I dropped drama and art and signed on for physics, chemistry, biology, and calculus. But for my fifth course, I chose creative writing.

I decided to pursue veterinary medicine. I wanted the adventures of James Herriot, driving around the countryside and mucking around in barnyards. But I worried that I was too slight to handle livestock. And caring for domestic pets—canaries and Persian cats—struck me as frivolous, not the elusive "real thing" that I was chasing. When I overheard a dorm mate announce that she wanted to be a doctor, her sense of purpose resonated with me. I decided to pursue medicine as well.

Of my three sisters, two became elementary school teachers and one a stay-at-home mother. I wanted a family too, eventually, and time to spend with it. I had no idea how it would all work.

In my first year of medical school at the University of British Columbia, we were divided into groups of five and assigned a cadaver to dissect over the year. On that first August afternoon in the anatomy lab, two dozen bodies lay face down on stainless steel tables with cloth sacks over their heads. We were introduced to the body gradually. Our first assignment was to dissect the upper back, supposedly the most impersonal part of the anatomy. Weeks later, we flipped the body over, and eventually we revealed the face. We cut, we identified, we sketched diagrams. We wrote the exam. The bodies were cremated. First year was over.

But it felt unfinished. There were other details on which we weren't examined—details I knew I'd remember long after I'd forgotten the divisions of the brachial plexus. How we were so moved by a Band-Aid crossing our incision path on our cadaver's forearm that we unanimously agreed to cut around it. The tattoo pigment accumulated in his lymph nodes, gathered from a faded inscription on his trunk, a name that we couldn't decipher. How we lifted his heart from his chest and held it in our hands, reverent and terrified; how his heart was the size of his fist, just as we'd been taught, but so much heavier. Those details could be acknowledged in writing, though. My poem was published: "Reflections on Seven Months with a Cadaver." American poet Mary Oliver, in her poem "Sometimes," gave three "Instructions for living a life: Pay attention. Be astonished. Tell about it." [1] I decided I would tell about medicine by writing.

I went on to do a two-year residency in family medicine at St. Paul's Hospital in Vancouver and then joined a private practice in Kitsilano. It was a practice filled with anxious professionals. One day, when yet another thirty-year-old woman came to see me because her hair wasn't as lustrous as it had been in her twenties, I realized that I hadn't gone through the rigours of medical training to spend my days reassuring the worried well. They were the equivalent of the Persian cats I hadn't wanted to see as a vet.

I wanted to care for sick patients who needed a doctor. I started working in Vancouver's Downtown Eastside and spent two years working at the BC Centre for Excellence in HIV/AIDS. But once I landed a position at Vancouver's refugee clinic, I settled in for a good decade.

The clinic was the real thing. Patients were suffering, and I had something to offer. The pathology was fascinating, and so were the stories. I adored my colleagues, deeply committed, generous people who were unconcerned with money or recognition. I was certain I had the best job of anyone I knew.

The American writer and theologian Frederick Buechner said: "The place God calls you to is the place where your deep gladness and the world's deep hunger meet."[2]

So, in that sense: yes, I had a calling.

3

As I drove the kids to school on my way to the clinic, winding along Dollarton Highway with the morning sun glinting off Burrard Inlet, my nine-year-old daughter told me about a mathematics contest she had written earlier in the week.

"I left one question blank," Saskia began. It was a confession: a perfect score was off the table. She didn't add up test scores; she worked back from 100. "But I did that because of how the scoring system worked. You got six points for a right answer, two points if you left it blank, and zero points for a wrong answer. I wasn't sure about the last question so I just left it."

I made her repeat that, making sure I had it right. Making a wild stab at an answer was worth less than no response at all? This wasn't the grading system I'd grown up with, which promoted doing one's best even if it involved guesswork. I was pleased that she would be rewarded for acknowledging what she didn't know. *If only we'd all pause to consider whether we truly know the answer to a question at hand,* I mused as I swung into the school parking lot. *And if not, take two points for keeping our mouths shut.* Over breakfast I'd read the comments on a CBC article about refugees, scanning the vociferous opinions that were ignorant of the basic facts of the system. I was dismayed by the misinformation and the arrogance that was posted.

After Saskia and Leif extracted their backpacks from the trunk, I turned the car and my thoughts toward the clinic. A medical student would be shadowing me this week. I was a clinical instructor in the Faculty of Medicine at the University of British Columbia. The refugee clinic was a popular elective choice, and most days I supervised a student or resident. I considered the recognition of one's limitations a critical component of physician training, albeit an uncomfortable one.

During my own two-year residency training at St. Paul's Hospital I had been assigned to a family practice for several four-week blocks, with callback every Thursday afternoon. It was an established practice at the intersection of two arterial Vancouver roads, Broadway and Granville, and a good group of doctors. I dreaded seeing the patients, though—mostly well-heeled, reproductive-age women—because I couldn't answer their questions.

Making a diagnosis and treatment plan on my surgery rotation or in the emergency room wasn't a problem, but patients in this clinic kept bringing up issues that weren't in any textbook. One couldn't interpret her baby's cries; another needed advice on dealing with strangers' remarks on her child's birthmark; the next had discovered her teenage son's porn collection. I was twenty-six, childless, and had nothing to offer on subjects that weren't in my medical library. I felt useless. I could only take a detailed history and call in my preceptor to finish the visit.

My preceptor and the other staff doctors took the entire clinic staff out for Christmas lunch that first year, between morning and afternoon clinics packed with patients wanting to be seen before the holidays. My preceptor paused during the meal and said to me congenially, "You know when we knew you were okay?"

I had no idea, but I was relieved they'd arrived at that conclusion.

"Remember that rash?" she asked. "The four-year-old with the vesicles on his legs who'd just come back from camping?"

I remembered. Yet another patient that had stumped me.

"When I asked what you thought it was, you said, 'I don't know,'" she went on. "That's when we knew we had a good resident."

The other physician agreed. "We don't care what you know," she said. "We care that you know what you don't know."

Now, a decade later at the refugee clinic, I was still keenly aware of the limits of what I could offer. Often there wasn't a satisfying answer to a problem. I used the traditional SOAP format for my chart notes: *Subjective, Objective, Assessment, Plan*. Often, the *P* could feel terribly inadequate. *Counselled* meant I'd dispensed words, five to ten minutes' worth. *Conservative management* meant I wasn't going to do anything yet. *Follow* sounded the most like a fail, although it was in fact a promise: *I will see you in my office, again and again, until you feel better.*

Doctors hear the God-complex jokes all the time, but I am well aware of my limitations. The practice of medicine teaches how very much is unknown.

The medical student who was shadowing me for the week was waiting in my office when I arrived at the clinic. We looked over the day sheet that had been printed and set on my desk. The morning's first patient was an elderly Bedouin woman, recently arrived from Syria. "I don't know anything about nomads," the student confessed.

We were off to a good start. "That's okay," I said. "You'll know something after the visit."

New learners often expressed anxiety about *cultural competence*, a buzz phrase in medical education. They worried that they would inadvertently offend a patient whose customs and beliefs differed from their own. I think of culture as a system of permissions, or, *How we do things around here.* The term *cultural competence* implies mastery, an expert knowledge of all these systems. Without immersing oneself in a culture for many years, it's impossible to appreciate all its nuances. American pediatrician and activist Melanie Tervalon suggests that we ought to strive for cultural humility instead.[1] That was what I taught my students.

When our clinic did a community engagement survey to assess satisfaction with our services, not one respondent complained of cultural insensitivity. This was not because the staff never made blunders, I assured students. It was because patients were forgiving when they recognized that practitioners came from a place of humility and goodwill.

Every year, I had to ask a Muslim patient to give me a refresher on Ramadan. *What are the dates? What are the hours of fasting? Who is exempt?* No patient ever scolded, "You've worked with refugees for ten years! Shouldn't you know this by now?" They were always eager to educate me.

I had made plenty of gaffes over the years. I'd complimented a patient from Myanmar on her shoes, only to have her remove them; the interpreter chided me: "Now she must give them to you." I'd routinely used a thumbs-up sign when delivering good test results to patients, only to learn that it was an extremely lewd gesture in Middle Eastern culture. I'd disgusted an Iranian patient when I passed him his shoes after his physical exam. "You're a scientist!" he'd said in a pained voice. Touching shoes, the epitome of filth, should have been beneath me. And those were the *faux pas* I was aware of.

"Just recognize that you don't fully understand the patient's context," I told the student worrying about the nomad, as we headed toward the waiting room to call her in. "And be curious!"

He nodded.

We passed the weigh scale, where a nurse was encouraging a little Somali girl in a long orange dress to stand straight against the measuring stick with her head level. Three sisters under the age of seven looked on, giggling, their teeth flashing white in dark faces wrapped in bright scarves. The mother undressed the baby, a pudgy infant with dark curls who craned his neck to watch the girls. "Wow!" whispered the student as we passed by. He looked excited, nervous.

The family struck him as exotic, I knew. They were too beautiful and unusual not to comment on. I'd felt the same when I started at the clinic, impressed by what was foreign. The differences in language, clothing, skin, and customs were too much to ignore.

In my early years of practice, I attended a refugee health conference where a speaker shared the words of Canadian anthropologist Wade Davis: "Indigenous cultures are not failed attempts at modernity, let alone failed attempts to be us. They are unique expressions of the human imagination and heart, unique answers to a fundamental question: What does it mean to be human and alive?" [2] The first words stung. Was I guilty of this? Was my delight in my patients' differences rooted in a subconscious interpretation of their failed attempts to be me?

I'd grown up with a church missionary calendar hanging in the kitchen, a new one every year. January's picture was a woman in Papua, New Guinea, with a baby on each hip, in the doorway of a hut with a metal roof. February showed a dozen African boys playing soccer with a ball of tinfoil. March was a group of Indonesian women washing laundry in a river. Every month we looked at a new picture of people on the other side of the planet who needed the things we had: food, soap, salvation, modern cars. As an eight-year-old I felt sorry for them; I felt lucky to be me. I hoped I hadn't carried this primitive thinking into my adult life.

Wade Davis' words challenged me to focus on something other than our differences: What made us human and alive? As a physician, seeing people at their most vulnerable, being privy to their deepest hurts and fears, I was afforded a little window into the human condition. Working at a refugee clinic offered me more clues as to what was universal about humankind. What did my vastly diverse patients share with each other, and with me? I'd determined a few commonalities over the years. We all loved our children with the same devotion. Everyone sought community of some sort. We all understood the language of kindness and humour. We sought purpose and meaning. No one escaped brokenness.

In the exam room, I sat facing the Bedouin patient, a tiny woman with white hair who appeared to weigh ninety pounds. She looked around the room with interest. The interpreter was seated to my left, and the medical student sat next to her, entranced. The patient looked at me with bright eyes, and I gazed back. She wore brown robes and had tribal markings on her face, dark blue geometric figures on her forehead and chin. I wore a navy suit and mascara. She didn't speak English, and I didn't speak Arabic. She was from the Syrian desert, and I'd grown up in the Pacific Northwest. We regarded each other with mutual curiosity.

The nurse had noted high blood pressure during the assessment at Welcome House. I gestured for the patient to push up her right sleeve and took the blood pressure cuff from its holder on the wall. She appeared frail, so I decided to forgo the complicated task of helping her climb from a step stool onto the exam table, and to take the measurement from where she sat next to my desk. The coiled black cord connecting the cuff to the wall-mounted sphygmomanometer stretched taut as I gently Velcroed the cuff around her arm. The room was quiet except for rhythmic puffing as I began to inflate the cuff. Suddenly, there was a loud pop as the cord, stretched to its limits, snapped from the wall, struck me across the torso and then dangled, tightly coiled again, from the patient's arm. I jumped. The patient looked up at me, and when she saw I wasn't hurt, she squeezed my arm and laughed out loud. So did I. And there it was, a foothold on common ground.

We spent the next half hour taking a proper blood pressure measurement, reviewing blood work, talking about her grown sons, and discussing her housing situation in Coquitlam. When I ushered her out after the visit, the interpreter said to me, "She wants to know if you have children."

"Yes."

"She wishes God's blessings on them."

4

IT WAS ALWAYS AWKWARD WHEN a patient requested "enough condoms for a month," and I was left to gauge whether to dispense two or forty-five. I'd given the patient in front of me—a twenty-three-year-old Kenyan woman—a generous handful of prophylactics in a discreet paper bag at her last visit, at her request. I'd encouraged her to consider a more reliable form of contraception, such as an IUD or hormones, but she declined. She'd had irregular menstrual bleeding on birth control pills in Nairobi and was reluctant to try anything other than condoms.

Now her period was two weeks late. Before I did the urine pregnancy test, I asked, as I always did, whether a positive result would be good news or bad news. The Swahili interpreter relayed my question. "Babies are always good news," said the husband reproachfully. "Gift from God." The patient, wearing a brilliant patterned pink tunic and matching headscarf, said nothing.

Minutes later, I broke the good news to them. "This is your fault!" said the husband. "We ran out of condoms but we had to wait weeks to get an appointment with you."

I looked at the patient. It was difficult to catch her eye. "Maybe this one is a girl," was all she said. They had three boys at home. The oldest was five.

Unplanned pregnancies in my patients always surged in the months after arrival in Canada. The cause of the fertility boost was unclear: the new-found privacy of one's own home, maybe, or physiological release after years of stressful living. Some patients were dismayed at the timing, concerned about the potential impact on finances and English class attendance. And of those that were pleased with the news, none had been on the recommended three months of folic acid to prevent neural tube defects.

I considered family planning an urgent issue. As well, most eligible patients had never had a Pap test or mammogram. I booked every woman for a clinic visit devoted to sexual health soon after her arrival.

It was two weeks since I had met the Haddads, and Junah had an appointment for such a visit. I saw her alone, with just the interpreter. She wore a navy coat, with a floral headscarf wound snugly around her tired face. Her birthdate in the chart had surprised me; she looked at least ten years older than forty. It was the weariness and the sag of the shoulders. I motioned for her to sit in the chair next to me. She glanced nervously at the tray next to the exam table, with the metal speculum placed next to a collection of swabs and slides. I eased into the visit with my standard questions.

The GTPAL score is an obstetrical method to compress a woman's reproductive history—fertility, miscarriages, twins, abortions, anguish, joy—into five digits.

G for gravida. "How many times have you ever been pregnant?" I asked Junah. Layth, Nadia, and Sami made the number three, at minimum.

"Six."

G6, I wrote. "How many babies did you deliver?"

"Three."

T for term, P for preterm. "Were they born on time, or early?"

"All three late!"

G6 T3 P0.

A for abortion. "What happened to the other three pregnancies?"

She described three first-trimester miscarriages.

G6 T3 P0 A3.

L for living children. I didn't need to ask her this one. That moment of drawing the 2, the curve devolving into a flat line when it should have been a symmetrical, buoyant 3, caught me in a way that the family's weeping at the first visit hadn't. Sami had been an integer, a whole number. The awful story was captured in a score that had been reduced by one.

G6 T3 P0 A3 L2.

I was always cautious about how I asked about contraception. The negative connotations of the accepted Western terminology contradicted the view of many of my patients that children were a divine blessing. Rather than "contraception" or "birth control," I referred to "family planning" or, better yet, "birth spacing."

Many of the couples I saw, particularly Muslims, quietly differed on how many children they wanted. Women sometimes returned to see me alone and request contraception that they could keep secret from their husbands; the nurse and I gave them injectable progesterone every thirteen weeks. One patient requesting clandestine contraception, a twenty-one-year-old Afghani woman with three kids, had explained to me desperately, "I want to go to school, learn English!" (Her husband came to see me months later concerned about his own virility: "Doctor, we've been trying for six months now, and no baby!")

Junah was forty, and it had been twelve years since her last pregnancy. I took a gamble. "What do you use for birth control?" I asked.

"Pills." She pulled a slim package from her purse. The graphic was soft pink and cream, the favoured palette of pharmaceutical companies marketing to women. It had Arabic script on it, Bayer's trademark cross in the corner, and "Gynera" in English.

I was relieved that Junah was using contraception. She had the dual risks of advanced maternal age and consanguinity. Pregnancy would be high risk.

"We don't have Gynera in Canada, but I can prescribe an equivalent," I told her, squinting at the tiny script on the back of the box. I was unable to even determine whether the list of active ingredients was in Arabic or English.

"I need a baby," said Junah, quietly, urgently.

I looked up at her, then at the interpreter.

The interpreter conferred with Junah. "She wants to get pregnant," she confirmed. "She wants a healthy son. Now that she is starting her new life in Canada, it is a good time."

"No pills," said Junah, taking the Gynera box from my desk

and dropping it into the garbage can. She smiled at me. It was clear that her mind was made up.

I laid out the issues as gently as I could. A forty-year-old woman, on average, only ovulated four times a year. Should she conceive, the risk of chromosomal abnormalities, such as Down syndrome, were greatly elevated by her age. The fact that she and her husband were first cousins contributed further genetic risk. I kept quiet about my concerns that her miscarriages and Layth's disability were due to consanguinity. Pregnancies in women of advanced maternal age carried higher risk of everything from pre-eclampsia to preterm labour, I concluded.

She tolerated my warnings serenely. "I need a baby," she repeated simply when I had finished. I realized that with Sami's death, the worst had already happened to her. She feared nothing.

The choice was hers, not mine. Not all physicians felt this way, it seemed. I'd had another patient in her forties who told her gynecologist about her wish to conceive a son. The specialist prescribed what the patient understood to be a prenatal vitamin. When the patient described the dosing to me—"Three weeks of the red vitamin, one week of the white"—I realized that it was an oral contraceptive pill.

"There are some things we should do before you get pregnant," I told Junah. "Some blood tests to check your health and to see whether you need any vaccines. You should take prenatal vitamins for three months before you try to conceive, to reduce the risk of health problems in the baby. And I'd like you to see Medical Genetics."

We waited while the printer hummed and churned out the requisition and prescription. I felt resigned. Junah looked elated.

5

A FAMILY DOCTOR TOLD ME ONCE, "It can be tedious seeing forty patients a day, but if one of those cases is interesting, it's worth it." We didn't see the usual lineup of coughs and prescription refills at the refugee clinic, though; something interesting came up hourly.

My eleven o'clock patient, an Iraqi man who had spent the past four years in Jordan, heaved himself onto the exam table and settled back, head on the papered pillow. I asked to look at his belly and he pulled up his green knit sweater, loosened his pants, untucked his checked shirt, and tugged that upward, too.

I'd seen thousands of abdomens, but I was taken aback by this one. It was riddled with six-inch scars that looked like graffiti, hurried purple strokes. The marks weren't from trauma or torture; they were surgical scars that were illegible to me.

If a Canadian-born patient were to lie on my exam table, I

could give a fairly accurate account of their medical story from their abdominal scars. A Pfannenstiel incision, a discreet line skimming the pubic area, suggests a Caesarean section. Three short, neat scars scattered over the right upper quadrant point to a laparoscopic cholecystectomy to remove a gallbladder. A one-inch line angled over McBurney's point in the right lower abdomen is almost always from an appendectomy.

But when I examined patients from the world over at the refugee clinic, surgical scars sometimes baffled me. I couldn't imagine what surgery could possibly have required an incision running from under the right ribcage, across the belly to the left lower abdomen. I didn't know what series of procedures would have resulted in a flank criss-crossed with red finger-length scars, or why an appendectomy scar would be five times the length I would expect.

The Iraqi man could tell me only that "the surgery was to stop the pain in my stomach." Like most of my patients, he had no medical records.

I examined his scars. I palpated them. I could not translate them. I ordered some blood work and arranged an ultrasound to provide some clues.

Detective work to piece together a medical history in the absence of records was routine at the clinic. The morning's next challenge was Layth. He stood up eagerly when I called him from the waiting room. He wore a fitted baby blue T-shirt with navy script emblazoned aggressively across the chest: NOT HERE TO MAKE FRIENDS. He beamed at me nonetheless.

My patients often wore curious things: tap dance shoes from the thrift store, clicking promisingly on the laminate flooring on the way to my exam room; a Justin Bieber backpack on a

Syrian senior in a three-piece suit; long johns in a cheerful print of moose and evergreen trees beneath the long black coat and slacks of an Iranian woman, revealed when I examined her swollen ankle.

The week before, an Afghani mother had brought in her daughters for assessment of their coughs. Although she wore a hijab, the girls, aged four and six, wore Western clothes. I asked them to remove their coats so that I could examine their chests. The jackets came off, and the sisters were wearing matching pink T-shirts featuring a prominent stylized image of a black bunny with a tuxedo bow tie.

There was no time for small talk about Layth's wardrobe. We had thirty minutes for an assessment of his developmental delay. I wanted to move us closer to a diagnosis and determine which investigations and specialist referrals he needed.

Layth sat next to his dad in my exam room, arm slung affably across Yusef's shoulders. "How's your new place?" I began.

Hani repeated the question in Arabic and relayed Layth's reply: "It's good. The neighbours have a dog. He hears sirens sometimes."

This was a situation where being unable to communicate directly was particularly frustrating. When engaged with an English-speaking patient, I automatically assessed diction, vocabulary, and rate of speech. A brief conversation could be rich with information regarding intelligence and mood. Layth's soft Arabic speech told me nothing, and it would be inappropriate to ask Hani's opinion of his IQ.

I took a detailed history of Layth's development from conception. Junah's pregnancy had been uneventful, Yusef told me, and the delivery uncomplicated. We went through

Layth's gross and fine motor skills, language acquisition, and social development.

"Floppy baby," said Yusef, rolling his head. "Hardly moving. When he was sleeping, like a frog." This was the classic description of an infant with low muscle tone lying on its back, hips abducted and legs extended. "But always very fat," he continued, poking affectionately at Layth's belly, encased in the T-shirt like a sausage.

Nadia, two years Layth's junior, had walked before he did. He was four years old when he took his first steps. "The week Sami born," said Yusef. "Good, because not enough people to carry three babies!" Layth didn't speak until age four; even then, his speech was unclear and he didn't speak a sentence for another few years. He had always had trouble following even basic instructions. He flapped his hands when excited.

I moved on to the physical exam. Layth's most impressive physical feature was his synophrys, or monobrow: his prominent black eyebrows were fused into a massive archless ledge. He had widely spaced eyes and a low hairline. He had prominent top front teeth, which he ground continually during the visit. His trunk was generously padded with fat, but he was thin elsewhere, particularly his fingers, which were extraordinarily long and slender. These were mildly unusual features taken individually, but as a constellation, with his developmental delay, they suggested a genetic disorder.

Given that Yusef and Junah were first cousins, I suspected he had inherited an autosomal recessive condition and received the same damaged gene from both parents. In recessive disease, if only one in a pair of genes is faulty, an individual is unaffected. But if Junah and Yusef had both inherited the same single compromised gene from their common grandfather, for example, and passed on that gene to Layth during the roulette of his conception, the pair could manifest as a devastating condition.

Layth had gone sixteen years without a formal diagnosis. Had he been born in Canada, he would have been assessed as an infant. This was not an uncommon issue at the refugee clinic, and it could make referrals difficult.

One of the most unusual afternoons of my career had occurred during a walk-in clinic years before, when five adult intersex siblings had turned up. They each possessed various combinations of male and female genitalia, which I carefully sketched into their respective charts. Raised in a rural South Asian village, they had never received medical care. Their parents had simply decided in each case whether to raise the child as a son or daughter. Some of the siblings did not identify with the gender selected for them. All of them felt that their condition restricted their ability to pursue relationships and to marry. Where to refer them? Urology? Gynecology? Endocrinology? Medical Genetics? I wasn't sure any specialist in Vancouver had experience with an intersex patient first diagnosed in adulthood.

However, no matter how difficult specialists typically were to access, they were always enthusiastic about the unusual cases we referred from the refugee clinic. A man from a remote South Asian village was diagnosed in Canada with a rare form of congenital dwarfism—one of only three families known world-wide—and went on to be presented at international medical conferences. When a patient was hospitalized with leprosy, three services—Infectious Disease, Dermatology, and Internal Medicine—fought to claim him as part of their turf. A woman with an arm deformity since birth was sent to the hospital's media department for photos prior to her surgery. Parasitology sent us a Christmas card once with little worms on it, to thank us for all the great specimens we'd sent them that year.

Patients were grateful for the specialized medical care. While they benefited from the increased interest and attention paid to their diagnoses, I reminded students that patients did not have the same enthusiasm for their conditions that we did. While the professional satisfaction of treating an unusual disease was undeniable, the patient simply wanted her suffering alleviated. No one wants to be the excellent teaching case or the subject of grand rounds.

I ordered a head CT for Layth and wrote referral letters to Medical Genetics and Pediatrics. Aside from a diagnosis, I didn't expect much to be offered. If his condition was genetic, there was no cure. I tried to gently probe Yusef's expectations.

Patients' hopes rarely meshed with what Canadian medicine could offer. I'd had a Somali patient with his arm amputated by an explosive weep with happy disbelief when I described a prosthetic arm. But over-expectations were far more common. A patient crippled by childhood polio was bitterly disappointed when an ambulance didn't bring him directly from the airport to the hospital to be cured.

"Layth going to school," said Yusef simply. "We so happy." Layth would be starting public high school in two weeks, with an aide. His settlement worker had connected him with the Ministry of Children and Family Development, which had made the arrangements briskly and as a matter of fact. There was no debate over whether he was an appropriate candidate for school. It made me proud to be Canadian.

6

PETE AND I WERE GETTING ready for work when he set down the iron, inspected his pants, and sighed, "Not these ones, too! All of my pants have grease stains across the thighs."

"So do mine!" I told him. "Grease stains, mid-thigh."

We puzzled over the consistent appearance and placement of the marks, and then we realized the cause. The range of the stains exactly matched the heights at which four-year-old Ariana planted her little hands when she grabbed us.

I'd been a mother for nine years, and during that time I had never gone into work wholly pristine. I'd had breast milk spit-up on my shoulder, crusted rice cereal on my shirt cuffs, teething biscuits cemented to my pant legs, apple juice splash marks on my shoes, and now a tideline of grease across my thighs. I wondered if I should resume wearing a white coat, but anything short of floor length would be inadequate.

I started work at nine. I got up at six. Even though we made lunches and laid out everyone's clothes the night before, we needed that much time to get all five of us packaged and delivered to our respective places of work and play in good spirits. I showered, dressed, and helped the kids pull on play clothes and school cardigans while Pete made breakfast. There was a flurry of smoothing hair into pigtails, stowing rain boots in backpacks, pouring coffee, and hunting for library books. At 7:30 AM, with the front door open in readiness for the five of us to brave the November chill and head for the van, I crouched in the front entrance hurriedly stuffing Ariana's hands into mittens.

I ushered her out the door, entreating her to pick up the pace as she dawdled down the walkway, stuffing pine cones into her pockets. Once in the van, I reminded her repeatedly to climb into her car seat, as I deposited backpacks in the trunk. I had read that children had no sense of urgency, that it was a waste of time to try to make them hurry; my years of parenting confirmed this. However, from time to time I couldn't resist trying to instill the importance of efficient routines. "Mommy and Daddy can't be late for work," I told Ariana urgently. "If we are, we could be fired!" Unlikely though that scenario was, the statement sounded sufficiently grim.

My words seemed to have an effect. I had her full attention. "They would set you on *fire*?" she asked with real interest.

We drove Saskia and Leif to before-care at their school. Then we headed over the bridge and into the city, where we brought Ariana to daycare. Finally, Pete swung by my clinic and dropped me off on his way downtown. I used the half hour before my first patient to review lab results and catch up on work email.

At two minutes to nine my colleague burst through the door, unstrapping his bike helmet. He was forty and single. His hair was a mess, he was out of breath, and he seemed exhilarated. "I woke up ten minutes ago," he announced. "I just rolled out of bed and out the door!"

Watching him hang up his reflective jacket and rummage in his briefcase for a granola bar, I could vaguely recall a life where my only real responsibility between waking up and presenting myself at work or school was to put on clothes. Now, I could hardly remember what it was like to show up at the office without feeling like I'd already done a full day's work. My colleague had the enviable ability to be single-minded. That was what I found most difficult about mixing medicine and motherhood: the diffusion of focus.

My work in refugee medicine was profoundly rewarding; raising three little ones even more so. The two had proven to be compatible. And yet at some point the efforts put into one required sacrifices of the other. There simply were not enough hours in the day for me to invest what I wished into both spheres. I had erred on the side of mothering, and while I did good work at the clinic, I felt that my career trajectory had been modest.

Caring for both patients and children was not easy. I'd attended a medical conference the year before where the presenter had flashed a list onto a giant screen, saying, "These are attributes of physicians that serve them well profession- ally: control; perfectionism; competitiveness; dedication; perennial caretaker; emotional remoteness." The audience had nodded and murmured in recognition. He had continued, "And these are the attributes of physicians that are liabilities in family life." He flipped to the next PowerPoint slide. It was an exact replica of the first. As the audience burst into appreciative, rueful laughter, I was struck by how neatly my domestic difficulties had just been explained. I'd often noticed that the very qualities that enabled me to do a good job at the clinic frustrated my efforts at caring for my family and our home.

My days at work were organized exactly as I liked them, from the length of patients' appointments to their medication lists to the position of the stapler on my desk. I interviewed patients, examined them, and ordered investigations. I didn't determine who walked in the door, but I managed every aspect of the problem once it was presented to me. My life at home was an unpredictable, distracted mess. Urgent requests and displaced items greeted me at every turn. I might be the one guiding the day in a general sense, but the thousand details were determined by three spontaneous children.

At the clinic, I took on challenging work, completed it, and turned to the next diagnostic puzzle. At home, I repeated menial tasks thousands of times while others undid them. The satisfaction of measuring performance by objective standards at work could not be achieved in the same way at home. I could pick up the faintest of heart murmurs, I could suture a laceration beautifully, I ran my clinics on time, but how do you grade yourself on raising a daughter well?

Like most physicians, I thrive on competition. It has always motivated me, and winning is powerful affirmation. But motherhood is different from the MCAT, pharmacology prizes, and residency applications. No one is going to come out on top, and comparing oneself to other mothers is futile and dangerous ground. The competitive mother after gold stars is the one no one wants to be around.

I wanted to be a great doctor and, even more, a great mother. But if the qualities of one could be the undoing of the other, it was no wonder my life felt like such a struggle some days.

Despite these challenges, I had work-life balance. It was precarious, something that I knew could be toppled by illness or an aggravating colleague or a newborn, but I rated my satisfaction with both career and home life as high. The philosophical and practical guidelines that I followed were these:

Accept that you can't have it all. At least, you can't have everything at once—but you can have a life that is rich and full and satisfying. I watched resignedly as other (childless) physicians at my clinic left to spend months working in Afghanistan and Peru. I was the mother who arrived late to the preschool Christmas potluck and set a box of Mandarin oranges next to the homemade cheesy noodle casseroles. I'd been meaning to replace my son's embarrassingly short school uniform pants for months. I couldn't attend a recent cross-cultural mental health conference because I was home with my daughter on Thursdays. But I had kind, secure children and what was arguably the most delightful patient population in the city. It was enough.

Be clear about your boundaries. Don't apologize for them. I worked part-time. I couldn't start any earlier than 9 AM due to school drop-off. I'd had potential employers rework schedules and change clinic start times when I told them my availability.

Don't compare your finances to others'. Leif asked me once, "Where do you and Daddy get money from?" He was taken aback when I explained that we were paid for our work.

All this time he had assumed we were going to work for pleasure and to help others. This pleased me to no end. I didn't want money to be the prime consideration in my decisions.

Every year the BC Ministry of Health puts out the "Blue Book," which lists the amount every physician in the province bills the Medical Services Plan. I'd perused it before, but no good came from seeing that my family physician-neighbour billed more than five times what I did. I started to gauge the wrong things in terms of money; how could I put a price on quiet days at home puttering in the yard with my four-year-old?

Say no. I considered this the most important skill I'd learned in the last five years. If I felt awkward saying no to someone's face, I'd say I'd consider their request. Then I'd say no by email. I didn't bother with reasons or excuses. I came across a quote from Dr. Gabor Maté's book *When the Body Says No* that I thought of almost daily: "If you face the choice between feeling guilt and resentment, choose the guilt every time." [1]

Write. I took ten minutes once or twice a week to document what had been memorable recently. This had a magical way of allowing what was important to rise to the top while the irritations of daily life drifted away, affording perspective.

Consider exhaustion the state of having given freely. One afternoon as I rounded the bend to approach the Second Narrows Bridge on my way home from work, the CBC's Rich Terfry on the radio and Ariana strapped in the backseat, I thought with dismay how overwhelmed with fatigue I was. I felt drained, spent, exhausted. Reflecting on these words, I realized that resenting what others had taken from me was passive and inaccurate. I had given what I had by my own choice. When considering Dr. William Osler's words, "Let each day's work absorb your entire energy and satisfy your widest ambition,"[2] anything short of collapsing into bed each night, completely spent, felt like a waste.

Travel lightly. I tried to apply minimalism to every aspect of my life. Visitors remarked on how tidy our home was, but the truth was that we had very little *stuff*. I decided early in my career to leave my part-time position at the HIV clinic to focus only on my work at the refugee clinic. We ate simply. Any commitments were carefully selected for a defined period.

Hold an annual general meeting to evaluate your life. Once a year, Pete and I hired a babysitter and took an evening to take stock of where we were at in every major area of our life: his work, my work, finances, church, where we lived, parenting, friendships. We identified what was working, what needed to change, and when we ought to re-evaluate. We liked to feel that our choices were deliberate; we didn't want to float up to our forties to say, "Huh! So this is how we live."

Find a great partner. Pete (who worked full-time in a non-medical field) was supportive, hands-on with the kids, and flexible around gender roles. We both made sacrifices. He was undoubtedly the linchpin to my contented state as mother-doctor.

I'd loved William Wordsworth's poem "Nuns Fret Not at Their Convent's Narrow Room" since I studied it in English 103, particularly these lines: "In truth the prison, unto which we doom/Ourselves, no prison is."[3] I was a mother in medicine by choice. I accepted any challenges and restrictions inherent to being a physician-mother, for that was exactly what I wished to be.

7

THE NEXT TIME I SAW Yusef it was November, the week before Remembrance Day. When I called him from the waiting room, he pointed proudly to the red poppy pinned to his coat. "I participate in the celebrations of my new country," he said through the interpreter. My own lapel was bare.

"Something strange happened last week," he said as we headed down the hall. He described how at nightfall the streets around his apartment complex were overrun with people dressed as ghosts and vampires, knocking on doors, with a sound like gunfire in the background. Hallowe'en was always confusing to newcomers experiencing it for the first time, without warning. A nurse had told me about one of our patients, hospitalized on the seventh floor of St. Paul's Hospital, who had asked politely when the fireworks began, "Excuse me, is there a war?"

My own neighbour had set up a ghoulish scene in his yard, to the delight of the kids on our street. RIP: REST IN PIECES read one sign in dripping red paint. I was grateful that such violence was so far removed from Vancouver that my kids found the sign funny, but I had a patient whose brother had been macheted to death, who had collected the body parts in a box. I'd always been sensitive to violence, but with each story I heard in my exam room, my tolerance sank. Hallowe'en is for dress-up, not gore, I'd tell my kids. I went trick-or-treating with a chicken, a nurse, and José Bautista.

Once Yusef had been briefed on Halloween, we moved into the reason for his visit. He wanted to donate blood. I double-checked with the interpreter that I'd understood the question correctly. "You've only been in the country for six weeks," I said. "What's the urgency?"

"I want to pay Canada back," he said. "And right now, the only thing I have to give is my blood."

"You can check with Canadian Blood Services to see if you're eligible to donate," I said. I found a pamphlet in the wall rack and handed it to him. He folded it carefully and slipped it into his back pocket, satisfied. I hadn't donated blood in years.

"Let's review your lab results," I said, turning to the computer.

Upon arrival, the Haddads had been offered the usual screening blood tests for HIV, syphilis, hepatitis, and anemia. The tests were often misunderstood by patients. Many assumed that the government and employers could access the results and use them as a basis for deportation or employment. Some thought that the authorities used the blood for experiments; this idea was bolstered by the multitude of tubes required to collect even the basic screening, which struck patients as excessive. Patients worried that they would be scolded or shamed for any infections. Despite these fears, and the fact that the tests were not mandatory, patients never refused them.

Screening for disease, an important component of primary care in Canada, was a novel idea for many patients. Most were used to accessing healthcare when there was a problem: pain, bleeding, deformity, disability. The concept of searching out asymptomatic disease, or risk factors for a condition that might manifest itself in the future, was a foreign concept.

"I'm not sick, but you want to find something wrong with me," Yusef had commented wryly when I recommended we add a test for diabetes and cholesterol to his initial blood work, based on his age.

It wasn't the first time I'd heard that accusation. After a normal routine breast exam, I'd recommended that my fifty-five-year-old patient have a screening mammogram. "Why?" she'd asked. "You said my breasts felt normal."

"There are limits to what I can feel," I'd explained. "An X-ray of your breasts can find even very tiny lumps."

She had been unconvinced. "Let's not go looking for problems," she'd said. "Bad luck."

She had a point. Mammograms often have false positives, and patients are called back for further testing that eventually, after provoking intense anxiety, proves to be nothing. Eighty-four women must be screened annually from age forty to eighty-four in order to prevent one breast cancer death.[1] While this NNS—number needed to screen—might be acceptable to physicians, my patients were less impressed by it.

Yusef's initial blood sugar test had been elevated, and

I'd asked him to repeat it. I looked up the most recent result: 7.3 mmol/L. "Your sugar is still a little higher than it should be," I told him. "Let's check your blood pressure."

I check blood pressure on almost every patient, in part as an excuse to touch them. It is therapeutic for patients, although the practice didn't come naturally to me. My parents weren't physically demonstrative. The Dutch cultural norm of greeting with three kisses on the cheek—right, left, right—was abandoned when the founders of my childhood community set sail for Canada on the *Groote Beer.*

When we practiced physical exams on one another in medical school, I felt awkward and timid. On the receiving end of my classmates' palpations, though, I noticed how much more pleasant touch was when it wasn't tentative. I learned to touch patients with purpose. "Grip the patient!" I told my own students now when I saw them auscultating a chest, left hand hovering uncertainly over the patient's shoulder. Touching patients establishes connection. It serves to comfort and reassure.

Yusef heaved himself onto the exam table, unbuttoned the cuff of his dress shirt, and rolled up his sleeve. His exposed forearm was covered in dark hair. I could smell cologne, faintly. I wrapped the cuff around his arm, Velcroed it securely, and began to inflate it. I inserted my stethoscope eartips and watched the wall-mounted sphygmomanometer. Using my stethoscope always reminded me of snorkelling: the mysteries just under the surface, the privilege of listening in, and the muffled noise of the outside world. It was a thirty-second vacation from the rush of clinic. The needle dropped steadily to 142 and then began to bob, as the pulse became audible. This continued until the needle pointed to 86, when its movement slowed and the pulse disappeared.

"It's a little high," I said as I released his arm and he rolled down his sleeve. "Same as last time. We'll check it again next visit."

"When I left Iraq I was healthy," said Yusef pointedly. "Canada has made me sick."

"Your blood pressure and sugars have probably been like this for a long time," I said. "It's just that we're learning about it now." I was careful not to slap a handful of labels on newly arrived patients. "You're not sick," I assured him. "These measurements are just a warning. They're giving you a chance to make some changes, so that you don't get sick in the future."

As we reviewed diet and exercise, I wondered at the practicality of the discussion. Health is already a low priority for most refugees, after more urgent issues like housing, employment, and learning English. With two kids starting high school, a wife attempting to conceive, and his insistence on paying Canada back, I didn't expect Yusef to be particularly concerned about preventing a hypothetical future health event.

I wondered how much he was currently affected by the trauma he'd experienced in Mosul. He hadn't told me further details of his abduction since the initial family visit, and I hadn't asked. It was a difficult line to straddle: ensuring that he understood that I was willing to hear the story, while giving him the space to decide whether to share it. Eliciting the story when the patient isn't ready risks retraumatization.

Some patients spilled every detail of their traumatic experiences to the first person in Canada who would hear it, often the nurse doing the screening visit at Welcome House. Some learned to use their stories as a kind of currency, to unlock services and sympathy. One Middle Eastern patient kept a slideshow of horrific images on his phone, set to music. Others kept their stories secret for years, even denying knowledge of how traumatic injuries had been sustained. A young African woman had casually asked my opinion about scars on her back, dozens of fine white horizontal lines laddered over her spine. I was at a loss as to how the markings could spontaneously appear. A year later she revealed that she'd been whipped; she didn't disclose why.

A few patients appeared remarkably unscathed by awful experiences. A Syrian politician who had had a cavalcade of thirty cars pull up to his home to arrest and imprison him for five years exuded such peace that I felt compelled to ask him about it. He told me with deep satisfaction: "Life is about the message. I had a message and for years I gave it to the people that needed to hear it. When I was jailed, they took away my freedom, my wallet, my health—but they couldn't take away my message."

Cultural attitudes toward past events differed, too. I'd asked a Myanmar woman once what she talked about over tea with her neighbours, also newly arrived refugees. "Do you talk about life in Canada, or the old days in the camp?"

She'd looked shocked at my question. "We talk about life in Canada. Everyone knows to talk only about our new life!"

An Afghani patient, on the other hand, had once recited a proverb to me: "One thousand years is not too long to hold a grudge." She, and others in her cohort, had had a very difficult time moving forward with a new life in Canada.

Over 80 percent of refugees exposed to trauma recover

spontaneously upon reaching safety.[2] Research shows that patients' mental health benefits from attention to basic needs, such as shelter, language acquisition, and the ability to work or attend school. And so I didn't press Yusef on his experience. I gave him an Arabic version of Canada's Food Guide and directions to Canadian Blood Services on Oak Street.

8

THE PATIENT WAS A YOUNG Iraqi mother. When I asked her how she was doing, she spoke so quickly that Hani couldn't keep up with the interpretation. Suddenly the patient stopped talking and dug in her purse for her phone. She stabbed at the screen with her index finger. She was going to show me a photo, I was sure of it.

This often happened at the clinic, and I never knew what I was going to see. Sometimes it was an album documenting the progression of a rash, blotchy red patches spreading over a torso. Once it was a picture of the patient in his previous life, standing in front of a grand home with an orange grove out front. And sometimes patients showed me something terrible: third-degree burns sustained during torture, or a crucifixion.

She passed me her phone, the screen filled with an image of dead bodies in someone's home. I looked at the picture like it was my job, because it was. It was part of caring for this patient. Something didn't make sense, though, and I automatically did a finger spread, zooming in, only to realize that the bodies were mutilated. I handed the phone back to her, and she looked grimly satisfied. The visit ended soon after. She didn't need anything else.

When I called Yusef from the waiting room a half hour later, the young Iraqi mother was sitting on one of the pews, and she blew kisses at me with both hands.

"I have burning," said Yusef once he was settled in the exam room.

"Where?"

"Everywhere." He gestured expansively at his arms, legs, and abdomen.

"What kind of burning?" I asked. "Tingling? Numbness? Pain?"

Hani explained these subtleties to Yusef.

He considered them. "Only burning," he said.

Almost weekly, Yusef checked in to the afternoon walk-in clinic with a similarly vague complaint: fleeting central chest pain while riding the SkyTrain; intermittent difficulty swallowing rice; excessive belching in the evenings. Each time, I took a thorough history, examined him, and ordered any necessary tests. Every time, the results were reassuring, and the problem migrated to another part of the anatomy.

I suspected that the diagnosis lay in a simple observation Junah had made at her last visit with me: "Yusef screams in his sleep." If I was going to ask Yusef about his mental health, I'd have to do it in a roundabout way, without reference to mood, crying, or worry. The stigma of mental illness, ingrained in Canadian society, is even greater in refugee-producing countries. Furthermore, most of my patients did not consider psychological issues to be part of the medical domain.

I started with my most proven access point to mental health assessment: "What time do you go to bed, Yusef?"

"Eleven o'clock."

"How long does it take you to fall asleep?"

"One or two hours."

"What are you doing during that time?" I knew the answer; I'd heard it a thousand times.

"Thinking. Thinking."

"Do you think about what happened in the past, what's happening in your life now, or what might happen in the future?" Worrying about one's daughter making friends in school was completely different than reliving a traumatic event or planning one's career.

"Always thinking about the past."

"Do you control your thoughts, or do the thoughts control you?"

He looked startled, found out. A confession: "Thoughts control me."

I patted the left side of my chest with the fingers of my right hand, twice. "How are your spirits?"

Every patient, well-trained by their ESL instructors, dutifully responded, "Fine!" when asked, "How are you?" Enquiring about someone's spirits while pointing at the heart, though, seemed to be universally understood as permission to divulge one's actual state of mind.

"No good," said Yusef quietly, after a pause. He pulled something from his back pocket, a folded brochure. It was for a local community program, and on the cover was a photograph of an elderly man with his head in his hands, and a consoling friend beside him. Yusef held up the pamphlet, pointed at the photo and looked hard at me. "Me," he said, his voice breaking. "Me."

There was a long pause. "Doctor, can you injure yourself by crying?"

"No."

He nodded, slowly. "Sometimes, when I cry so hard, it feels like something might break inside."

He told me what had been done to him by his abductors. He described an assault on the body intended to break the spirit, ensuring he would never recover. The account of inhuman acts was so degrading that I would never allow the details to leave the exam room. I wouldn't enter them into the electronic medical record or debrief with colleagues. I wouldn't share even a basic account, stripped of patient identifiers, with Pete or my closest friends.

In the future, when someone at a family dinner would make conversation by asking me, "What's the worst story you've ever heard at the clinic?" this would be the one I'd think of, and I'd be enraged that someone could enquire so lightly about trauma, wanting only to be titillated, while reaching for ketchup.

I was turned away from the computer, facing Yusef squarely. I sat with my feet hooked on the stool footrest, my hands on my legs, shoulders loose. I listened. Over the years at the refugee clinic, I'd cycled through various responses to patients' stories of trauma. The gamut I had run was wide: voyeuristic fascination with the horrific details; avoidance of patients' pasts when I became overwhelmed by my powerlessness to change them; feelings of deep shame over being human; detachment, where I could hear a story of torture while noting that it was lunchtime, debating whether to order the black bean soup or the cucumber and gorgonzola sandwich at the deli. Eventually, I simply focused on absorbing patients' stories. I came to believe in the healing power of bearing witness to suffering, a belief borne partly out of results, partly out of resignation.

When I was first at the refugee clinic, young and green, I wanted to prescribe treatment for a Congolese patient's parasite; she wanted to tell me about being raped by her neighbour. As she spoke, slow and soft, I panicked because I didn't have a plan. None of the usual medical responses applied, in that brisk bullet point way that physicians love—a prescription, procedure, referral. There was no solution. What was I to say when she finished her story?

Now, a few years later, I taught my residents that it was presumptuous to even think there existed a fix for something of such nature or magnitude. No one shared a story of intense suffering and expected to be offered a solution. As difficult as it was to just listen—to accept one's impotence—it was enough. And so I said nothing. When Yusef finished speaking, I said only, "I'm sorry to hear how much you've suffered. No one deserves to be treated like that."

After disclosing a horrific story, patients always did one of two things: they apologized, or they thanked me. Yusef apologized.

That night, two girls walked into a bar. A bistro, actually, a block from the Park Theatre on Cambie Street, where *The Grand Budapest Hotel* was playing. And we weren't exactly girls anymore, with six kids and two thousand patients between us. The bistro had a bar, though, and my friend Erin and I had a half hour till show time.

She ordered a beer and I had a whiskey sour. The place was packed, Friday-night noisy. I poked at the ice in my glass with a straw, and Erin told me about a case from her practice in Comox. The server approached with a tomato and bocconcini salad, a glorious trifecta of tomatoes, basil, and cheese with the balsamic drizzled artfully across the plate. I expected her to pass by, but she stopped and reached over to set it down between us.

"That's not ours," I said, regretfully.

She looked confused.

"It's not ours," I said again. "Not unless someone ordered it for us."

She took it back, apologetic. "Your face just lit up when you saw it," she said.

"It does look delicious," I admitted. We laughed, she brought it to the couple a few feet up the bar, and Erin and I returned to our drinks and conversation.

Ten minutes later, the waitress approached with another tomato and bocconcini salad. She set it down in front of me. It was *déjà vu*, except this time the bartenders and another server paused to watch, smiling.

"Someone ordered this for you," she said. We stared at the plate.

"The guy that was sitting at that table over there," she said, gesturing behind us. "He ordered this for you." I turned, and he was gone, leaving just a crumpled napkin and the bill folder on the table.

Our show was about to start, but I enjoyed every slice of Roma tomato, every pale oval of cheese, every basil leaf, and with each bite I thought happily: *A stranger bought me a bocconcini salad, anonymously, simply to delight.*

I'd recently read a description by American essayist Phyllis Theroux of an ecstatic experience where she watched the morning sun light the cockleburs next to a sleeping porch. This was an experience from which she drew strength later:

> Could it be, and this is the question of a speculative, unmarveling adult, that every human being is given a few sights like this to tide us over when we are grown? Do we all have a bit or piece of something that we instinctively cast back on when the heart wants to break upon itself and causes us to say, "Oh yes, but there was this," or "Oh yes, but there was that," and so we go on?[1]

A few weeks earlier, I'd seen media images of captured Iraqis before and after execution by militants. I saw their faces and hands. I struggled to grasp that humans treated one another that way, and I couldn't make sense of it. Then I read an article in the *Guardian* about men being raped in war, and it fit exactly with my experiences at the refugee clinic. A person, deliberately, severely damaged by another person. Multiplied by a thousand people, over a thousand wars. And then today, Yusef's story.

Months later, when my heart wanted to break upon itself and I was desperate for a small reassurance to hold onto, I remembered that story—the one about the guy who bought the girl at the bar a bocconcini salad.

Oh yes, but there was that. Humans do that, too.

9

THE WEEK BEFORE CHRISTMAS, VANCOUVER received the season's first big snowfall. It was only a few inches, but everything was transformed by a soft, homogeneous glow. I took public transit to work—the SeaBus, the SkyTrain, a few blocks by foot in snow boots.

In every other clinic I've worked, patient attendance is influenced by the weather. Patients stay away if it's too sunny, too wet, too slippery, too hot. Not so at the refugee clinic. Refugees have overcome such massive obstacles that inclement weather is a negligible deterrent, I suppose. Sure enough, every patient booked that morning showed up. I was the one who arrived late.

Between patients, Hani told me about her first snowfall after arriving from Somalia. How unbelievable it was, how beautiful. She put her hand over her chest, trying to convey her amazement. "Everyone who comes to Canada and sees snow for the first time, they never forget that," she told me in her soft voice. "Never."

I enjoyed seeing patients' responses to seasons in their new country. "We're celebrating Christmas like real Canadians," said the first patient, an Iraqi father of two. "I even took my kids to see that white guy in the red suit."

The next patient was an Ethiopian grandmother who had arrived in Canada that fall. She lived in Surrey and walked her grandchildren to school every day.

"Do you celebrate Christmas?" I asked as I peered into her left ear with the otoscope.

"Not in the past," she said through the interpreter. "But now that we're in Canada, we celebrate what Canadians celebrate. So we will have Christmas this year."

I was excited for her. "Will you have a Christmas tree?" I asked.

"What's that?"

The third patient was a fifty-five-year-old Iranian woman with diabetes. She was due for bloodwork, and as I filled out the requisition form she asked hesitantly if she could wait a few days before going to the lab. She lowered her voice and said carefully, "Because I'll be celebrating a . . . holiday this week."

"You mean Christmas?" I asked.

"You too?" she gasped.

Yes, me and most of the country, and none of us feared persecution for being found out.

Mid-morning, Yusef and Junah came in. "We couldn't rebook to come in the New Year," Yusef explained, "because we had to see you before Christmas to give you this." Junah pulled a small wrapped gift from her purse. It was a bracelet, a slender silver band with a geometric motif engraved at the centre. I was moved, and not just because they'd braved the icy sidewalks to deliver it.

Yusef said a little speech, thanking me for what I'd done, the support and the kindness. "You helped us when we were new in the country, in trouble." I felt professional gratification that they were satisfied with my services; I told them with sincere emphasis that it was my pleasure to care for them. As I ushered them out the door I'd already forgotten their gratitude.

"That was a beautiful speech," said Hani after they left.

I looked at her and I thought, *Yes, yes it was beautiful.* I'd heard these speeches before, though, thanking me for kindness, and I felt embarrassed to be thanked for dispensing something that cost me nothing: no extra education, no honing of skill, no effort. I'd rather be thanked for diagnostic prowess or a deftly performed procedure. But I extended kindness to patients habitually, with an extra measure when I had nothing else to offer. *You shouldn't need to visit a clinic for kindness*, I thought. There should be an abundance of it free for the taking as you move through daily life.

Later that week, I sat in *my* doctor's office, in the chair tucked right next to his desk. This was the first visit that I didn't sit casually on the exam table with my legs dangling over the side, the first time I hadn't come in for something routine like a vaccination or contraception, where we'd talk shop and I'd ask about his daughter, a medical school classmate. This time, I was here about a disastrous ending to a second-trimester pregnancy.

He knocked on the door, stepped in, and gave me a long, sober look as he slowly closed the door. He sat down.

I couldn't look at him. He sat in silence. Finally, I forced myself to talk, exhausted, crying, despairing. He listened. He leaned over his desk, arms folded on it, looking down. Eventually I glanced at him, and his face was flushed. His eyes were damp. I realized that he was moved by my distress; I was completely taken aback.

Over the next few weeks, as I celebrated Christmas and rang in the New Year with my family, I repeatedly thought back to our encounter. The memory of him sitting there, seemingly with all the time in the world, fully present, saying little but moved by my situation, was an enormous comfort. His kindness was more dear to me than anything he'd done for our family over the years, even his delivery of my daughter.

I saw him in follow-up three weeks later. The visit was such a solace that I was certain I was being extended divine kindness; my doctor was the unwitting priest. What a profession! What power! I imagined, longingly, that I could extend the same gift to my patients.

And I realized with horror that this kindness, which had affected me so profoundly, was the very one that I used unthinkingly in my own practice, that I dismissed as a personality trait, a last resort for patients for whom I had no medical therapy to recommend. I had been wielding something powerful without any respect for it.

Back at work, I was determined to be conscious of what I gave to patients, and to receive what they returned to me. An elderly Congolese patient with severe osteoarthritis had found a French-speaking family physician near her home. She made a short, thankful speech, and this time I didn't dismiss the gratitude as grossly disproportionate to what I'd done for her. "Every visit, I felt better just to see you," she said. She hugged me; I felt very slight. She pressed her cheek against mine, and I could feel and smell her hair. "Don't forget me," she said through the interpreter. "Come visit my home."

Weeks later, I saw my doctor again. I was doing much better, and he seemed mystified as to why I'd come. I wanted to check in, I explained. I could see him trying to figure out what I wanted from him. He offered a medication, and I declined. He offered a different one, but I didn't want any medications. He asked again why I'd come. He had no idea, I realized, how therapeutic his presence was. The simple answer was this: all I needed, quite literally, was to see the doctor.

I saw him in the wild, once, months later. I came out of my clinic on the way to lunch and looked up from putting my stethoscope in my purse to see him hurrying along the sidewalk. It was a grey day, wet and blowing. His white hair was flying, his head hunched down. He wore a brown leather jacket and a red plaid scarf looped once around his neck.

It was disorienting, seeing him as a civilian. I realized then that I had never seen him in outerwear. In fact, I had only seen him under the strictest of conditions: in dress pants and tie, in an eighty-square-foot exam room, between nine and five. This was, as birders say, a lifer.

I felt as comfortable in his exam room as I did in mine. When he took my blood pressure, squeezing my arm, he was close enough that I could smell his laundry detergent. He wore button-down shirts with his initials monogrammed on the pocket. He recommended novels and told stories of his travels. He always ran late, but he never glanced at his watch when he was with me. At the end of the visit he would turn on his heel and hurry down the hall to the next patient. I chose not to think about the others.

When he delivered terrible test results that time, and my husband and I were heartbroken, I learned later that he had gone to a community meeting that same night to speak against a proposed neighbourhood casino. Our devastation hadn't followed him out of the office—of course it hadn't—and the realization stung.

When his notice of retirement came in the mail soon after, he thanked his patients for allowing him to share in their joys and sorrows. Not illness and health—joys and sorrows. He had had a front-row seat to mine. Mine, and those of a couple thousand other patients. This was a form letter, one of a massive mailing; my sinking heart was one of many.

It felt awful, being forced to acknowledge the nature of our relationship: it was business. He was a professional friend, really—supportive, non-judgemental, reliable, accessible, and an excellent secret keeper, because he was paid to be. Who wants to acknowledge that they purchased care, paid for intimacy? The truth, though, was that he gave me what I couldn't get anywhere else.

I was embarrassed whenever I suspected a patient felt a strong personal attachment to me. I was willing to be appreciated for my medical skills, but I felt distinctly uncomfortable receiving anything resembling love. The obligation I felt to reciprocate in kind was in complete violation of my professional identity. And yet, my attitude toward my own doctor was one of devotion, and I expected nothing in return. He'd already given enough for a lifetime.

I'd had three complaints about me brought to the clinic

manager in almost a decade. All were in response to my efforts to discharge patients from the clinic to family doctors in their communities, three-zone SkyTrain fares away, after a year as my patient. Moving patients along was clinic policy.

The first patient sent a letter, run through Google Translate to render the Arabic into English, pleading for "continued care under the prestigious auspices of the clinic, by the human being Dr. Martina Scholtens." It would have been delightful if it weren't so urgent. He dismissed any reassurance that he could get the same services—better, even—closer to his home. It wasn't the service that he wanted. It was our relationship.

Once when I called Yusef from the waiting room, and we were friendly and laughing as he gathered up his backpack and umbrella, I saw another patient across the room, watching us. From the look on his face, I knew I'd been found out; I wanted to turn his face away. I could see his expression: confused, disappointed, processing that what he was to me wasn't special. How to make him understand that though our relationship wasn't, in fact, exclusive, none of it was a lie, either? How, when I hardly understood it myself?

10

DURING MY RESIDENCY TRAINING AT the family practice office at Broadway and Granville, I had been amazed at the gingerbread houses, chocolate gift baskets, and wine that piled up on the counters during the Christmas season, as well as the tokens of appreciation that flowed into the clinic year round.

Gift giving was an unusual event at the refugee clinic. The patients were typically of modest means; even bus fare was often an issue. The gifts that did arrive, though, were memorable. An elderly Afghani woman brought me a cardamom pastry made by her son, a baker. A mechanic gave me four blue air valve caps for my car tires. A Vietnamese couple brought me a straw hat with a message woven into it, which they declined to translate and I chose to assume was a positive one. A family whose mother I had treated presented me ceremoniously with a polished red apple. And I treasured the jewelry I had received from the Haddads, making a point of wearing the bracelet when I knew they were coming to the clinic.

This list might be delightful, but the truth was, receiving gifts from patients made me uncomfortable. It was a distinctly personal exchange in what I took pains to keep a professional relationship. I was conscious of the financial sacrifice involved for people struggling to pay rent. Sometimes I was given a token of gratitude for a result to which I contributed nothing. The cultural nuances of gift giving could be tricky to navigate.

When I was in the exam room, though, and the patient reached in her purse for a package, I learned to focus on one thing: respecting the meaning of the exchange to the patient. If I disliked feeling beholden after accepting a present, perhaps this was a taste of what the patient had felt for months. Maybe gift giving was a realization of the patient's independence that we had worked to foster, a move away from the sense of obligation and deficiency that can accompany receiving help.

After eighteen months at the clinic, I told an Arabic patient that he needed to move on to the family doctor he'd found in Richmond. He reluctantly agreed, but said that he needed to come back for one more visit, to bring me a parting gift. I told him that was thoughtful, but unnecessary. He insisted. I protested. I relented when he finally said, forceful with frustration, "You don't need a gift. But I need to give one."

At the end of a visit, a Myanmar woman handed me something wrapped in a plastic shopping bag. It was a brilliant pink, hand-woven skirt. I promptly tried it on over my pants. It was a perfect fit. As I thanked her, overwhelmed with how kind the gesture was, but also how unnecessary and costly, she repeatedly asked through the interpreter if I liked it.

When she had left the clinic, I pulled the interpreter aside and asked if it was appropriate for me to accept the gift. It was so generous, when all I had done was provide routine care.

She shook her head before I had finished explaining my hesitation. "You must accept it!" she said emphatically. Gripping my arm, she said quietly and firmly, "The Karens give gifts to people who they feel in their hearts are looking out for them."

I had tears in my eyes, because she said so simply what we strove to do in medicine, particularly for the most vulnerable patients at our clinic.

More embarrassing than accepting a gift was inadvertently requesting one.

Hundreds of Karens, an ethnic minority from Myanmar, had come through our clinic over a five-year span. They were accomplished weavers and soon after arriving in Canada they resumed working on their looms. They wore skirts and scarves in a fine weave, with intricate patterns and gorgeous colours. I particularly admired the bags that both men and women wore slung over their shoulders.

I finally asked Win, the Karen interpreter, where I could purchase such a bag. She had come into the exam room with a soft knock for me to sign her day sheet. She immediately looked excited. "What kind do you want? Zippers, to put lots of things in, or bag, or sling?"

I described the bag my patients usually carried, a simple tote. "Where can I buy one?" I already felt awkward; I could see exactly where this was heading, and it was too late to stop it.

"What colour?" she asked.

"Red and white," I said, remembering a particularly beautiful one I had seen a few weeks ago.

She started to thank me. "So many patients ask me if they can bring you a bag! But I didn't know. My sister, she asked me last week if she could bring you a bag! Thank you! Sometimes we use four colours. What if it is red and white and black?"

"Any colour is good."

"I will make it for you."

"No!" I protested. "Then I wouldn't have asked you!" I explained how I had searched online for a vendor, hoping that the Langley Weavers and Spinners Guild would offer them for sale. "Where do you sell them?" I asked.

"My house!" Win exclaimed. The interaction ended with her slightly bowing, hand over her chest, thanking me for the opportunity to make me a bag.

The next time she came to the clinic to interpret, she delivered not one, but two bags. Of course, reimbursement was out of the question.

Weeks later, I thanked her again for the bags, and told her that I thought of her every time I used them. She nodded vigorously and said in a serious voice, "I think of you all the time, too."

Sometimes I was recognized for work that I didn't do.

When I did a routine breast exam on an Iranian patient, I discovered an abnormality. I arranged some investigations. The patient was distraught, and no amount of discussion could calm her. The imaging confirmed a suspicious lesion, and a biopsy was organized. It came back benign.

She came in for the results a week later. When I gave her the good news, she began to sob. She briefly buried her head in her husband's shoulder, and then pulled out her cell phone and made a series of calls. All the while, via the interpreter, she asked me repeatedly to confirm that she didn't have cancer.

Then the thanking began. Profuse thanksgiving, to me. The interpreter could hardly keep up with the flood of appreciation. The gratitude made me uncomfortable, and I tried in vain to deflect it. At one point the patient uttered the first English phrase I'd heard from her: "I love you!" They finally left, clasping my hand on the way out.

When I came back from lunch, there was a package of chocolate pastries on my desk. I suppose that what I ought to have done was to store up this appreciation, undeserved though it was, and dole it back to myself to salve my wounds if next time, as the messenger, I got shot.

My favourite gift came from the Prairies, was given out of a misunderstanding, and was very difficult to explain to my family when I pulled it out of my briefcase at the end of the day. I had cared for an Iraqi family for almost a year, parents and four children, all of whom I'd seen regularly. One of the adult sons was a dentist, and was working toward his Canadian professional credentials. He needed to travel to Saskatchewan for an exam, he emailed me, and his dad was going with him. They'd need to cancel next week's appointments.

"No problem," I emailed back.

"Want anything from Saskatoon?" he asked.

"Some wheat?" I joked. "Have a good trip."

A few weeks later, I called the dad in from the waiting room. He cradled a Bulk Barn plastic bag on his lap. I started to sweat.

"What kind of wheat did you want?" he began, through the Arabic interpreter. "Because we went to four different stores, and said, 'Our doctor wants some wheat,' and at every store they asked, 'What kind of wheat?' We didn't know, so I hope this is what you wanted."

He passed me the sack and waited anxiously for my reaction. It was fluidly hefty. I looked inside, and there were several bulk bin scoops of hulled, unmilled wheat kernels.

We had long since passed the point of no return. "This is perfect," I said. "Thank you so much."

After the visit, the interpreter couldn't help herself. "Why did you ask him for wheat?" she asked.

"Because they went to Saskatchewan," I explained. She had immigrated to Canada a half dozen years ago; this ought to make perfect sense to her.

She looked at me blankly.

"Saskatchewan is famous for wheat," I continued, lamely. "Here, watch what happens when I do a Google Image search for 'Saskatchewan.'" She looked over my shoulder as my screen filled with scenes of golden wheat fields receding to a point on the horizon, under wide blue skies.

"Oh," she said dubiously. "I had no idea."

11

THE CLINIC LOST THE FEDERAL funding for its trauma program, a critical service for refugees who had experienced terrible events. I was dismayed by the decision, worried for my patients' well-being, and frustrated by the dismissal with which mental health services so often seemed to be treated. I wrote an appeal for its restoration. I worked on it for a week, in the evenings, after the kids were in bed.

I began the article with a litany of horrors that I'd seen at the clinic. I knew the names of everyone I described.

> I've seen an Iraqi mother disabled by a car bomb, and a journalist who was tortured with electrocution in an Iranian prison. I've cared for a Somali family whose newborn babe was flung to the ground and killed by rebel fighters, and Congolese

women who were forced to watch the executions of their husbands and sons. I've met Afghani and Pakistani women who were threatened with acid or death as they walked to school or work.

I appealed to empathy:

And still I watch as resilient and resourceful patients find a home, learn English, and seek employment. But for some, the trauma they have suffered continues to torment them. They relive horrific events through nightmares and flashbacks. They experience continuous fear, mistrust, and hopelessness. Sirens, police, or loud noise trigger panic. Psychological pain manifests as crippling physical symptoms. They mourn for and worry about family left behind. I see children who hurt themselves, mothers crumpled by shame for being raped, and fathers who cry when left alone.

I appealed to pragmatism:

Someone in that state cannot learn a new language, gain employment, or develop social networks. Adjustment to life in a new country is challenging enough when attempted with optimism and energy; it is next to impossible for someone whose psychological reserves have been completely drained.

These patients require intervention to achieve a level of peace necessary to function. Medication offers some benefit, as does primary care, but connecting the patient with a trauma counsellor is essential. Counselling enables the patient to process past events, achieve respite from psychological pain, and move forward with life. I've depended on Vancouver's trauma counselling services for my patients, and my colleagues and I are now forced to cobble together treatment plans as best we can from the limited resources that remain.

I voiced my frustration at mental health getting short shrift, again:

> Mental health should not be an add-on, the icing on the cake of medical care. It is foundational to the care of the patient. Stabilizing mental health ought to precede, or occur alongside, diabetes management, hip replacement, and prenatal care—not act as an optional part of patient care to be tackled at the end of the list, should there be leftover resources.
>
> The word *patient* has its roots in the Latin *patiens,* meaning one who suffers or endures. That is what I seek to do as a physician at a refugee clinic: to relieve suffering. With this population, I need mental health services to do it.

I submitted the article to two national newspapers. There was no response. I widened the net, sending it to local papers, news blogs, and medical journals. Only one deigned to reply, with a polite rejection.

I couldn't believe it. Was it poorly written? Was the issue too narrow and specific? Or—and this idea upset me most of all—did the editors know that it would bore the Canadian public? The lack of interest in publicizing the issue was a stinging second blow.

At the clinic, we triaged the patients in need of counselling and directed the most urgent cases to the Vancouver Association for Survivors of Torture. The others would have to wait, supported by their physicians, while we searched for more resources in the community. Finding counsellors who specialized in trauma, offered interpretation, and were accepting new clients was next to impossible. The list of patients waiting for care continued to grow. The most prevalent diagnostic codes at the clinic were for depression and anxiety.

Over the past months, I'd determined that Yusef met the criteria for post-traumatic stress disorder—PTSD. Details gleaned from his visits and from Junah's offhand accounts of life in their Surrey apartment led to my diagnosis. His abduction and torture in Mosul, and Sami's death, intruded into his daily life as flashbacks and nightmares. He went to great lengths to avoid reminders of his past. If he saw a dark blue sedan similar to the vehicle that his abductors had used, he froze until it passed out of sight. When he walked to get groceries, he made an elaborate detour around the neighbourhood parks and playgrounds with soccer pitches, fearful of a reminder of the after-dinner game he'd enjoyed with Sami in the final moments of their former life. He couldn't bear being near the water's edge and avoided the beaches for which Vancouver was renowned. He was hypervigilant, insisting that Layth and Nadia stay indoors when they weren't at school. He was easily startled and angered by something as benign as a slammed door. His sleep was poor.

I'd read once that an ideal story—dilemma, crisis, resolution—could be represented by punctuation marks: ? ! . It struck me that Yusef's story was the reverse: a peaceful life disrupted by horror, with no resolution: . ! ?

"Your nerves are tired," I told Yusef one morning in January. He nodded warily as Hani repeated this. "Humans are only built to withstand so much," I continued. "If you try to lift something very heavy, you'll hurt your back. In a similar way, there are limits to the suffering that people can endure. If it's too much, damage is done."

This was how I approached mental health, avoiding clinical, stigma-laden terms like *depression* and referring to *suffering* and *nerves* instead. "I'd rather have cancer than depression," a patient had wailed once, devastated with her diagnosis.

"Aren't you contributing to the stigma by avoiding the correct terms?" a psychologist friend challenged me at one point. I did introduce the proper terminology, eventually, after the initial sensitive conversations had been had. But in cautiously broaching the subject of treating Yusef's PTSD for the first time, I didn't want to risk alienating him with jargon he might instinctively resist.

"All of my patients are refugees, and many have experienced awful things," I told Yusef now. The torture prevalence among Iraqi refugees was 56 percent.[1] "Many of them describe what you've told me: nightmares, constantly checking that the door is locked, feeling like they can't control their thoughts." I could see disbelief on his face, then relief.

"I think I am crazy," he confessed in a soft voice.

"You're not crazy. What you're experiencing is a normal response to what happened."

We sat quietly. "I am confident that you can be well again," I offered. "There is no quick fix, but I am very hopeful that you can feel better again."

Tears ran down Yusef's face. There were medical differences of opinion on offering patients tissues. One camp encouraged it as an empathic gesture. The opposing view was that the message implicit in an offered tissue was, *Stop crying!* I took the middle ground by placing the tissue box in a conspicuous location, at arm's reach from the patient, where he could serve himself. Yusef did not take a tissue. Neither of us made an effort to stop his tears.

"There are a few options for treatment," I went on. I always provided these in the third person; this degree of separation seemed to offer patients some objectivity and make the choices less overwhelming. "Some people choose to wait and see. Sometimes, with time and settling into their new home, the symptoms resolve on their own." Yusef had been in Canada for only four months.

"Some people get relief from medication," I continued. This risked sounding horribly pat—writing a prescription to treat torture like you would an ear infection. "A pill can't undo what happened to you. I wish it could," I said. "What medications can do, though, is help your stressed nerves to rest, so they can heal. This takes time. You would have to commit to taking medication daily for at least six months." Yusef said nothing to this.

"Some people find it helpful to see a counsellor," I went on.

I could see him about to protest, and I knew what his concern would be. "You don't have to talk to the counsellor about what happened in the past, unless you want to. A counsellor can focus on how to feel better in daily life." He looked unconvinced. The concept of confiding problems privately to a trained professional was foreign to most of my patients.

"Studies show that the best results happen when medication is combined with counselling," I concluded. I waited for his response.

He didn't hesitate. "No pills," he said. "No counsellor. Just you."

Torture involved loss of trust, a speaker had said at a refugee conference I'd recently attended, and patients were healed by re-establishment of trust. I might not be a psychotherapist, but I had excellent rapport with Yusef and I recognized the value of it.

I nodded. Today, I was just floating the idea. I hadn't expected Yusef to do anything more than listen to it. I'd lost count of the patients who'd asked me months later, "Doctor, remember that pill for stressed nerves that you told me about?"

I gave him an Arabic handout on PTSD and offered some simple coping strategies. "More walking outdoors every day," I said. "Less time reading Al Jazeera online." I'd been taught that the most powerful words a doctor could say to a suffering patient were the ones I said next: "I want you to come back and see me in a week."

"One week," he said, slipping his arms into his coat sleeves. "One week."

12

THE HADDADS HAD BEEN IN Canada for five months and I had not seen Nadia, the fourteen-year-old daughter, since the initial family visit. Twice I'd reserved an appointment slot for her when her parents and Layth were due to come in, but both times she hadn't accompanied them. "Nadia at school," her parents had said simply.

I was pleased that she took her studies seriously. Furthermore, I knew healthy teens typically did not prioritize visits to their family doctor, but I wanted to have at least one visit alone with her. I asked Hani to call her directly and book an appointment with me.

This afternoon she'd been waiting alone on one of the church pews, phone in her hand and backpack at her feet. I'd asked the family medicine resident who had joined the clinic for the month of February to assess her. Nadia had given an unexpected history of epilepsy. Like virtually all my patients, she had no medical records. She was on no medication and her physical exam, as reported by the resident, was unremarkable.

"You're saying she's faking it?" asked the resident. I leaned against the counter in the chart room, eating my bagged lunch at 2:30 PM and considering what she'd just presented to me. Nadia waited for us in Room 146.

"No, I don't think this is malingering or Munchausen's," I said. I didn't believe that Nadia was faking symptoms or harming herself for medical attention. "Conversion disorder is when psychological stress manifests as neurological symptoms, such as blindness or paralysis."

The resident looked confused, and I didn't blame her. Conversion disorder was a rare phenomenon, and I hadn't seen any cases as a medical student or resident. I recalled one portion of one lecture covering conversion disorder in my medical training. It was memorable because the psychiatrist proposed that people miraculously healed by preachers at revival meetings were in fact simply having their conversion disorders reversed.

At the refugee clinic, though, I'd seen a half-dozen patients over the past year who responded to stress with impressive neurological symptoms. All of them were Iraqi.

One developed right-sided paralysis whenever he spoke to his elderly father in Baghdad. He'd been run through the stroke protocol at the emergency at his local hospital twice, both times resulting in a normal head CT and a shrugging neurologist.

Another had a Bell's palsy that recurred when the news reported a surge in violence in her home country. She'd come in with a drooping right eyelid and half of her mouth frozen in a downturn. A few days later she'd spontaneously recover.

I suspected that Nadia, whose seizure-like activity began upon the death of her brother Sami in Mosul two years ago, was our latest case of conversion disorder.

"How do you want to work this up?" I asked the resident. Conversion disorder is a diagnosis of exclusion—you must rule out other causes first. I agreed with the resident's plan for blood work, a head CT to rule out structural abnormalities, and an EEG to analyze the electrical activity of the brain.

I accompanied the resident to the exam room.

"Hi, Nadia." She was seated as far back in the chair as was possible, the smooth wrap of a pink hijab framing her face. She wore a thick application of eyeliner, skinny jeans with a small deliberate rip over each knee, and Adidas sneakers. She stared at me with frank curiosity, as Muslim girls often did. I was a novelty, I knew: a female physician in a pantsuit with loose hair.

"This doctor told me you've been having some trouble with collapsing and losing consciousness," I went on, nodding at the resident. I waited for the Arabic interpreter to relay this. "There are several possible causes. Let's start with some basic tests, and we'll see from there."

She managed the smallest possible nod.

"How's school?" I asked, while the resident completed the requisition forms.

"Okay." Whispered.

"What grade are you in?"

"Nine."

I could not imagine the challenges of navigating public high school as a recent immigrant with limited English skills.

"In Canada, doctor visits are not just for when you're sick," I offered.

She waited.

"You can see a doctor about other things, too—trouble with friends, having a boyfriend, feeling worried or sad, your sleep. You can come to the clinic with questions about your body or your period."

She was frozen in her chair. Then, without taking her eyes off me, she said a few quick words in Arabic.

"She doesn't have a boyfriend," said Hani.

My young patients often had misconceptions about Canadian social behavioural norms, assuming sex and substance abuse to be far more common than they are. If their culture endorsed abstinence, I worked to normalize it. "In Canada, some teenage kids have sex. Many don't. Choosing not to have sex is a healthy choice," I said. "If a man or boy wants you to do something that you don't want to, tell them no," I went on. "It's your choice, and you can say no." I was conscious of the vulnerability of my young female patients, and tried to have this conversation with each of them.

While Nadia said nothing in response, I could tell I had her full attention. I was sure she'd gotten more from this doctor visit than she'd bargained for. She looked shocked, but not displeased.

When I saw her again a month later, the results of the seizure investigations we'd ordered were normal. So were those ordered by the two different emergency doctors she'd seen in the meantime; both had been copied to our clinic.

Nadia seemed ambivalent when I gave her the results. She continued playing with a strand of hair. Both emergency consult notes indicated that paramedics had been called to her high school when she had a seizure. I asked her about this.

"I'm very embarrassed when an ambulance comes to the school for me," she said through the interpreter. "Everyone looks at me."

"I can see from the emergency doctor's note that he arranged a neurology consult for you," I told her. "And the second time you went to the emergency they set up an appointment with a cardiologist." I made sure she had the details for those appointments.

During the entire visit, at the back of my mind, I'd noted that something was different about her. Suddenly I realized what it was. "You're not wearing your hijab!" I said.

The headscarf was gone, and gleaming black hair hung to her mid-back. She tried to look nonchalant at my exclamation, but she couldn't hide a small pleased smile. She spoke to Hani.

"Her parents said that because they are in Canada now, she can choose whether to wear the headscarf."

Junah, I realized, had made a different choice for herself.

"At the last visit, you said she could ask you about her body," Hani continued.

"That's right."

She went on to describe vaginal symptoms that sounded like a yeast infection.

Before I could ask her to undress, Nadia thrust her phone at me. "There's no need for an exam," said Hani. "She took pictures."

On the phone's screen was a macro shot of a vulva.

"There's more than one," said Hani. "Scroll through!"

There was an entire album of Nadia's perineum. I hardly

dared to handle the phone; I was acutely aware that I was a few swipes away from sexting her entire address book.

"I can give you a prescription for Canesten," I said, "Please delete these."

When I saw her next, the cardiology and neurology reports had been added to the growing list of reassuring results. Patients were never as pleased to receive normal results as one would expect. A normal finding meant that their question hadn't been answered, which was frustrating. Some patients interpreted a negative test result as the medical system denying the existence of their symptoms, calling them a liar.

Broaching the subject of conversion disorder—suggesting to a patient that her symptoms were due to psychological distress—was always a sensitive task. I started by asking Nadia for her ideas on the cause of her fainting spells.

"They're psychological," she said simply. "I'm full of loneliness." She'd seen a half-dozen doctors, holding the answer the entire time, and not one of us had thought to ask the question.

We talked about connecting with a counsellor. I suggested anxiety-reducing medication. We reviewed sleep and exercise.

I ended the visit with my standard question: "Anything else I can do for you today?"

Nadia hesitated, looked down, and asked quietly, "Could you help me find some friends?"

13

OFTEN TURNED TO GOOGLE IMAGES to help supplement instructions to patients whose English was limited. I'd pull up a picture of prunes for the constipated patient, or a humidifier for parents with a coughing baby. A few words typed into the search box and the screen was populated with helpful images.

Patients that I'd seen often over the past year, an elderly Iraqi woman and her adult daughter, came to see me about the mother's shingles. She had terrible pain to her right trunk and as part of her treatment I advised that she apply lidocaine ointment to the affected area. The ointment worked best when an occlusive dressing was applied over top, but Saran Wrap was a cheaper alternative.

They were not familiar with Saran Wrap. Cling wrap? Plastic wrap? A see-through cover that could be stretched over food?

Miming pulling the wrap from the roll and wrapping a sandwich didn't help.

I turned to the computer and typed in my search terms. Mother and daughter leaned forward and looked expectantly at the screen. And then, multiple images of naked women bound in cling wrap appeared. I quickly turned the monitor away, but not before these two conservative Muslim women had been confronted with several seconds' worth of pornography.

This possibility had never entered my mind. Was this an established practice about which I was extraordinarily naive? We were all horrified, but I was the only one who blushed, and this, with my profuse apologies, seemed to amuse them. They made a sly reference to the incident at every visit I had with them after that.

Since then, it felt like a gamble to search even seemingly innocuous terms in front of patients, and I began to discreetly turn the monitor out of the patient's line of vision for a preview when I needed an image.

And then a Nepali-speaking family came in with a boy who had olecranon bursitis, an inflammation of the elbow. I advised icing it—with a bag of frozen vegetables, for example. They were confused, and I turned to my computer, screen carefully angled away. But they gathered around and watched over my shoulder. What could I do? I would have to chance it.

Bag of frozen vegetables, I typed. I couldn't think of any way that this could be abused, but I'd been wrong before. I held my breath. The results came up.

Peas and carrots. Oh, sweet relief. Nothing more than peas and carrots.

Communication with patients was always a challenge.

Eighty percent of clinic visits required interpreters. Patients spoke Arabic, Farsi, Swahili, Oromo, Spanish, French, Nepali, and a dozen other languages.

I was effectively and unfortunately monolingual. As a Canadian, it embarrassed me to request a French interpreter. When I took government-mandated Grade 10 French in British Columbia, I didn't have the slightest inkling that fifteen years later I'd be a physician to French-speaking Africans. If only I had learned how to ask about chest pain or bowel movements, instead of memorizing all the items one would bring *à la plage*, and the gender of a hundred fruits and vegetables.

Farsi or Arabic would have been more useful than French. I had investigated language courses at UBC and the local community colleges, but couldn't find any offerings that fit with my schedule. I had acquired few foreign language skills over the years despite constant exposure; I was focused on the medicine and the linguistics were just the backdrop to my work.

When seeing Spanish-speaking patients, *sangria* was one word that I heard regularly. It was usually buried in a long descriptive passage by the patient, and while I waited for the English version, I thought of a chilled red wine beverage with brandy and floating citrus slices. Finally, I asked the interpreter why the word kept cropping up. *Sangria* meant bleeding, it turned out, and my pleasant reveries had been completely at odds with the experiences patients were recounting. I think I may even have been smiling while someone described a hemorrhage.

According to a demonstration video we watched at a staff meeting, the interpreter ought to be seated behind the physician's left shoulder. Eye contact was to be maintained between doctor and patient; the interpreter was to function as a kind of unobtrusive machine, providing literal phrase-by-phrase interpretation. It didn't work quite like that. Sometimes the interpreter came with a large personality, extra commentary, or cologne that couldn't be ignored. We would compete for the attention of the patient, whose gaze would oscillate distractedly between us. Having a third party in the room could make it difficult to develop rapport with the patient.

Although I could never know for certain what was said by the interpreter, I needed to have reasonable confidence that the dialogue was being conveyed accurately. The regular interpreters were excellent and I trusted them. Sometimes I'd work with someone new, though, who would relay my carefully detailed instructions to the patient in five words. Or the reverse: my one-word answer would be interpreted to the patient in an excited tirade lasting minutes. Some interpreters had such strong accents that I misunderstood their English. One of the Swahili interpreters pronounced *angry* and *hungry* identically. I went through a painstaking history trying to sort out why my patient was angry all the time but it turned out he couldn't stop eating.

Literal translation was helpful for medical details, but sometimes the more nuanced meanings behind my questions were lost. When I asked whether a patient was sexually active she considered the question carefully and replied, "Usually I lie quite still." I stopped asking, "What brings you in today?" when one too many patients responded, "SkyTrain." When it came to patient stories, most interpreters used cultural interpretation, listening to the patient's entire story and then retelling it to me with cultural explanations. Sometimes I preferred the literal interpretation. I wanted to hear that a Somali woman's anger at those who killed her newborn was "like an animal chewing on my insides." I didn't want a Westernized description.

Patients had to be matched to interpreters of the appropriate sex and ethnicity. Most women, particularly Muslims, were reluctant to share gynecologic complaints through a male interpreter. A subtler challenge was appropriately pairing an interpreter to a patient with regards to ethnicity. We organized a Kirundi interpreter for a patient from Burundi. The patient was Hutu and the interpreter was Tutsi. While this distinction was invisible to me, they instantly recognized each other's ethnicity and refused to proceed with the visit.

Shared backgrounds with interpreters could cause confidentiality and disclosure issues, though, especially within a small refugee community with a limited pool of interpreters. An Ethiopian woman refused an interpreter for her visits because she was terrified that her HIV diagnosis would be leaked to the African community in Vancouver. I wondered how likely an unmarried Karen woman with pelvic pain was to disclose sexual activity when the interpreter sat in the church pew behind her every Sunday, or a Muslim with liver disease to reveal alcohol consumption when the interpreter was wearing a hijab herself.

Often the interpreter was beloved by the patient and became a confidant. Sometimes the interpreter supplemented the patient history with information from personal interactions in the community—at the mosque or grocery store. One of my patients, an elderly Vietnamese man, complained of poor vision. I was trying to establish the nature, severity, and progression of his symptoms when the interpreter cut in: "Doctor, I will tell you a story his granddaughter told me at church. He went to the grocery store this week to buy a birthday cake for her. He walked up and down the aisles until he found a large cake display."

She went on to describe how the patient selected a small, rectangular cake. It was light brown, and he assumed it was chocolate-flavoured, his granddaughter's favourite. As he was having some difficulty seeing the product clearly, he patted it gently with his hands. Through the plastic wrap the cake felt firm, cool, and moist. Pleased with his find, he made the purchase and carried it home.

He set it on the centre of the table in the dining room and went in search of birthday candles. As he rummaged in the kitchen drawer, his daughter entered the room and asked, "What's that slab of pork doing on the dining room table?"

With this exchange, the interpreter violated every rule in our staff educational video on professional interpretation. It was useful information, though. I decided my patient's visual problems warranted further workup.

14

SHE HAD A GARDEN THE size of my exam room, the patient told me through the Karen interpreter, appraising my eight-by-ten-foot office. I had been nosing around with my questions, curious, trying to understand the mysterious daily life of the depressed Myanmar mother sitting in front of me. I'd asked about plants, and she'd perked up. What was she growing? Mustard, pumpkins, and four kinds of eggplant. She'd started them all from seed as soon as the grey Vancouver winter had lifted and the days began to warm. The plants had grown this big: she held her hands a few inches above the exam table. It was the most animated I'd ever seen her.

"When she goes outside every day and sees that things have grown, she feels good inside," said the interpreter.

I understood. My own garden was a wild West Coast mess of sword ferns the size of small cars, mossy boulders, and drifts of cedar droppings like soggy orange feathers. Puttering in the yard for an hour after dinner was the perfect antidote to a day at the clinic. It was silent, except for the hum of boats motoring up Indian Arm. The work was manual and repetitive, and my mind could wander; gardening was meditative.

Results in the yard were blessedly tangible. American writer Michael Pollan described gardening as "ways of rendering the world in rows."[1] It was true: after the chaos of clinic it was a relief to engage in a pursuit where I could impose order. I decided what went where, and whatever threatened the plan I raked, weeded, and pruned, with visible and immediate effects. Measureable progress was directly proportional to the work I put into the project. Such were not the ways of medicine.

The temptation when I headed out to the yard was to focus on what needed fixing. I deadheaded the hydrangeas, scraped away moss, and swept the walkways. I had to make a conscious effort to focus on what was remarkable, to fuss around the rhododendron with its huge pink blossoms and take a cutting for the kitchen table. I tried to do the same at work and in life: to avoid focusing on what needed a solution, and to celebrate what was in bloom.

While I enjoyed being industrious, the real events in the garden—like the clinic—happened independent of me. I was, at most, a facilitator. When I stepped away from patients or plants for a few weeks, all sorts of interesting and surprising things occurred in my absence. Things were never as I'd left them. Both gardening and medicine were organic, messy, and unpredictable. Both had inherent vitality, a life of their own. This satisfied me deeply.

I was a permissive gardener. When I discovered cedars spontaneously sprouting in a corner of the yard, two inches tall and several shades brighter than their parents, I accommodated them. I weeded around them, thinned them, and cut back the salmonberry bushes so that they'd have more light. "Look how well my grove is doing," I'd tell Pete, who'd humour me with a glance in their direction. I had a similar approach to patients. I enjoyed puttering and discovery.

The pleasure of gardening—especially on days at home with my daughter—was sometimes sullied by my own speculation that it might be indulgent. Setting out slug bait felt frivolous when my patients were so traumatized by war experiences that they dissociated in English language class when they heard a siren. There was a wait for my patients to see me at the clinic, and here I was raking leaves. I was so acutely conscious of the needs of our patients that sometimes I was convinced that clinic work was the only activity worth my time.

I felt differently, though, after I read the United Kingdom's *Project on Mental Capital and Wellbeing* report.[2] It includes an evidence-based list of five simple daily habits for mental well-being, which are likened to five daily servings of fruits and vegetables and recommended to every person in the UK:

1. **Connect.** With the people around you. With family, friends, colleagues, and neighbours.
2. **Be active.** Go for a walk or run. Step outside. Cycle. Garden.
3. **Take notice.** Be curious. Catch sight of the beautiful. Remark on the unusual.
4. **Keep learning.** Try something new. Rediscover an old interest. Take on a different responsibility at work.
5. **Give.** Do something nice for a friend, or a stranger. Thank someone. Volunteer your time.

The report, the result of a two-year study involving over 400 international experts, concluded that making these activities a part of daily life could have a profound impact on people's happiness. This resonated with my professional experience. New Year's resolutions and doctor recommendations usually revolved around physical fitness—losing weight, eating well, and working out. It was harder to be specific about pursuing optimal mental health, and therein lay the beauty of the concise, practical list. With some intention, these five items could be seamlessly woven into most people's daily routines with little cost in terms of time or money. I wanted a prescription pad stamped with the list.

The recommendations crystallized a few things for me personally as well. The checklist validated taking time during the day for pleasurable pursuits, such as gardening. Knitting while Ariana napped, bringing a book along to the beach, or fiddling with a camera setting during lunch all included several of the five happiness-inducing habits. Now I could articulate why tucking away pockets of time for those activities during the day was not wasteful. It might literally preserve my sanity.

As well, the list explained why a day at the clinic was inherently satisfying, whereas a day at home with the kids required effort to produce the same sense of well-being. My work at the clinic ensured that I connected with colleagues and patients, took notice of the details of others' lives, learned continually, and gave to others. I ticked off four of the five mental health boxes just by going through my day. I checked off all five when I hunted for free parking and walked eight blocks to the clinic.

When I stayed home with the kids, few of those five activities occurred spontaneously. When I followed the path of least resistance, a length of time at home seemed to naturally tend toward isolation and inactivity. Most of my days at home were pleasant, but only because of the work I put into making them so. While at-home mothering easily held its own in terms of isolated blissful moments and long-term gratification, my state of mind at dinner time was sometimes one of defeat. "Go for a walk," Pete said when he got home from work and sensed such a mood. "Go walk in the woods." We lived near Wickenden Park, a dark, still forest with footpaths winding through it. A half-hour alone surrounded by cedars, huckleberry bushes, and bird calls never failed to calm me. Just as my patient had said, going outside and seeing that things had grown made me feel good inside.

"Junah is happier," Yusef remarked offhandedly the next morning as I refilled his prescription. I'd asked after the family, as I always did. "She didn't say that. But she must be, because over the past week she's filled the apartment with plants."

15

"Guess how many times neighbours have come to visit," commanded Junah.

I guessed that it was exactly as often as I'd dropped in unexpectedly on my own neighbours. "Zero."

She looked taken aback by my certainty. "Yes! No one has come for tea."

"They probably think they're being polite by leaving you alone. Try inviting them." I appreciated Canadian reserve, but Junah looked indignant.

Few patients were immune to loneliness. Sometimes I was tempted to connect two isolated patients with similar addresses, a friendly matchmaking service to combat loneliness. Patients needed to be part of a community, not just to fill the void of friends and family left behind but to be distracted from rumination about the past. Friendship offered an opportunity to practise English and learn the culture. Patients needed friends to feel Canadian.

I wished the public knew how important small gestures could be. When I heard the stories of little kindnesses that patients told me, I wanted to broadcast them. "I was walking with groceries, heavy bags, when the bottom dropped out of one," Yusef told me. "Potatoes, apples, cans—all rolling on the street. Then a car honked, and it was my neighbour! He helped me gather my groceries and drove me home in his car." The pride with which he related this suggested that it was about more than practical assistance. He'd been recognized.

I'd read a newspaper article about one of my Syrian patients. He described his new life in Burnaby with an anecdote about how he'd tripped and fallen on the sidewalk. Strangers had rushed to help him up. "Just like Damascus," he'd said with satisfaction. Stories like these moved me more than anything else I heard in my exam room.

I encouraged patients to connect with others, but I understood why it was so difficult. The language barrier was significant, as were cultural differences. In English classes, specific language groups stuck together. Mothers were intimidated by the other women clustered together at school pickup. The idea of joining the local recreation centre to swim or work out was often inconceivable, particularly to women.

Some patients did take the initiative, reaching out and exploring, but they were the exception. "I had my son's friends from college over for lunch on Sunday. An African and an Indian," an Iranian man told me. He was fascinated by Vancouver's diversity. Several of the Pashtun men from

Afghanistan instantly recognized Canada for the playground that it is, cliff jumping in Lynn Canyon, taking road trips, camping in the wilderness, and reporting their exploits to their incredulous doctor.

My patients weren't the only ones who were lonely.

On the face of it, a day at the clinic seemed social. I saw patients, one after the other, from nine until four, with a break for lunch. Most of my patients were well known to me. I'd get caught up on their lives—school, family, work. "How are your spirits these days?" I asked almost every time. It didn't get much more personal than that. It was just me and the patient, our knees almost touching, in a small exam room with the door closed and an interpreter behind me.

I left work after a day of this, drove the five minutes to pick up Ariana from preschool, and began the commute to Deep Cove. Suddenly I'd be ravenous. I'd ask Ariana what was left in her lunch box and she'd hand me some carrot sticks and cubes of cheddar from the back seat. Ten minutes later, around Grandview Highway and Nanaimo Street, I'd bottom out, utterly exhausted. The idea of having to shepherd kids through mealtime and bedtime chores felt impossible.

If Pete wasn't away on business, I came home to sous vide salmon and curried cauliflower, and we divided up the after-dinner work. If he was travelling, we'd eat the Costco lasagna my daughter put in the oven when she came home from school. Then I oversaw homework and lunch making, brushing teeth and laying out school uniforms for the next day.

I cut corners. I picked the bedtime book with one sentence per page. I moved up the bedtimes of the kids too young to notice. I wanted the noise to stop, even the singing. *They're getting shortchanged*, I'd think, *but I'll make it up to them later in the week.*

For years, I'd seen patients Monday, Tuesday, and Friday. Mid-week I was home with my youngest, grateful that Deep Cove was off the beaten path. We couldn't see our neighbours from our place. Standing at the kitchen sink, I could see a stand of waving cedars, the gunmetal grey winter waters of Indian Arm, and the dark bulk of forested mountains rising from the opposite shore. The solitude was perfect. No play dates, thanks. No community centres or meeting for lunch, either. I might be up for something on the weekend, but it took until Saturday evening to recover from Friday afternoon's walk-in clinic. I needed a respite from human contact, and I preferred as much solitary time outside the clinic as three kids could give me.

I'd forget, though, that seeing patients wasn't at all a substitute for catching up with friends over drinks. At the clinic, the topics of conversation, the confidences, the complaints—they were all one-sided. There was pleasure in seeing patients, but really, it was business.

I'd never have believed I would have three kids and eight hundred patients and feel lonely. But my work drained me to the point that all my spare time was spent trying to recuperate. Pete wanted to have people over more, and to vacation with other families. I had always imagined a noisy, boisterous home with friends and family coming and going, but with my work commitments, I didn't have the psychological reserves to make it happen.

My quietest sister lent me Susan Cain's book *Quiet: The Power of Introverts in a World That Can't Stop Talking.*[1] I had never recognized the challenges that my introversion brought to clinical work. Cain advises creating as many restorative niches in daily life as possible: "Introverts should ask themselves: Will this job allow me to spend time on in-character activities like, for example, reading, strategizing, writing, and researching? . . . [If not,] will I have enough free time on evenings and weekends to grant them to myself?"

No, and with three kids, no.

I had an epiphany. Clinical work's patient lineup exhausted me, and my social life was extremely limited because I needed stretches of alone time to recharge from work. I had to reverse this. I needed to implement more solitary time at work, and more people-time after hours.

So I gave up my Friday clinic. I'd worked Fridays since I finished residency. Now I finished the week with administrative work and other projects instead, alone in my organization's secret library. Just me, a row of computers with access to our clinic's electronic medical records, shelves of journals on pediatric nutrition, and a yellowing poster on Boolean operators.

I'd known since my residency training that I couldn't see forty patients a day, five days a week. I found it hard to do half that. Maybe it was that my patient demographic, with their trauma histories and multiple barriers to care, were particularly challenging. Or maybe it was the demands of three kids. Maybe our clinic needed to use a different model of care. Maybe an office with some natural light and a view of the North Shore Mountains would help. There were probably other changes I could make to bolster my psychological fortitude and soldier on, even thrive, in this setting. But to start, I reduced my work hours devoted to direct patient care.

After the switch, I had no regrets. Before, I felt like I spent everything at the office. Now I was making regular small deposits into my psychological savings account. I had the feeling of having extra pocket money. I heard the promising jingle of spare change.

16

AN OVERSIZED PINK UTERUS FLANKED by a matching set of ovaries was projected onto the wall. Eleven Myanmar women gazed at it, paper plates of cake balanced on their laps. As I began to explain the anatomy, one of them abruptly walked up to the screen, spread her arms wide, and clapped a hand over each ovary. "I know this," she said, quiet and proud. "I know this!" The others murmured and nodded. She had been a health instructor at their refugee camp.

The nurse and I had organized this women's health group visit for the new Myanmar arrivals who had been attending our Vancouver clinic over the past few months. They were Karens, an ethnic minority who had lived for up to twenty years in remote camps along the Thai-Myanmar border. None of them were familiar with cervical screening or mammography, and most of their pregnancies were unplanned. Teaching them as a group, we reasoned, would be much more efficient than the individual counselling we were currently doing.

And here they were, eating snacks in our clinic's meeting room, a collection of women aged eighteen to seventy-eight who'd taken the bus in from Langley together that morning. I felt like a hostess, responsible for the event's success and concerned that the guests enjoy themselves; I was relieved that they'd shown up at all. These were considerations foreign to a typical clinic day in my office.

That nervous feeling—that I was on unfamiliar ground, outside the comfortable routine of one patient, one exam room, twenty minutes—was the first suggestion that moving all of us into this new context might result in something unexpected.

Our experience to this point was that the Myanmar women were particularly pleasant patients: uncomplaining, compliant, deferential to a fault. Consequently, eliciting any kind of medical history was a real challenge. Repeatedly I found myself seated across from a slight, smiling woman in a bright woven skirt, with just a hint at a problem, doing the medical version of twenty questions. I worried that I'd miss a diagnosis because the history depended almost completely on me; I wasn't sure a patient would divulge a symptom like severe right lower quadrant pain unless I enquired about it directly.

But here as a group, with an interpreter, the women were transformed. They interrupted our presentations with comments and anecdotes. They asked questions and made jokes. There was a continuous soft running commentary the entire morning, and the atmosphere was congenial, even festive.

Susu, the interpreter, had come to Canada as a Myanmar refugee herself ten years earlier. She interpreted at clinics and hospitals across the city, sometimes disregarding the rules and transporting patients to appointments in her own car. She interpreted the sermon on Sundays at the church the Karens attended. She wouldn't call me by my first name, but surreptitiously paid for my lunch one day when we found ourselves at the same neighbourhood restaurant.

The nurse showed a slide with an image of a heap of packaged condoms in a rainbow of colours. There was laughter and discussion in the Karen language. Susu relayed the joke: "When someone handed those out at the camp we took a lot, because we thought it was candy!"

The nurse passed around an IUD, and the women closely examined the tiny T with long trailing strings. A discussion among them ensued. They looked concerned. "They're wondering," said the interpreter, "whether their husbands might become tangled in the strings. Trapped. Perhaps even injured." We trimmed the threads for future demonstrations.

As I explained the procedure of mammography, a woman raised her hand and asked slyly, elbowing her neighbour, "What about women with very small breasts—do they still need this test?" Giggling and more nudging ensued, and I realized that some jokes are universal.

I went on to explain the purposes of cervical screening. A hand went up, waving urgently. I paused. "She says," explained the interpreter, "that she needs that test. She must have it, right away." There would be a chance at the end of the morning to have that exam, I informed her. Two more hands shot up. In the end, every woman in the group wanted a Pap test that morning.

Once we'd finished the teaching, I distributed evaluation forms. Most of the women weren't literate even in their first language, so we'd kept it simple: four statements for the interpreter to read out, and a choice of circling a happy or sad face to demonstrate whether the respondent agreed. "We'd like to know how to improve this visit," I said. "This is anonymous. There's no need to write your name on the paper."

"But they want to," the interpreter relayed back to me. "They insist."

She read the first statement: "I liked the group visit today."

"Yes!" the women responded in chorus. The interpreter explained again that the answers needn't be shared. The women continued to cheerfully voice their affirmative responses to each question. When I reviewed the evaluations later, sure enough, all eleven respondents had given us a perfect score.

Each participant then had an opportunity to meet briefly with me one on one, so that I might answer any questions, and review contraceptive and screening needs. I'd expected that I could meet with each individual in the corner of the room, while the others visited and had more tea. But the other women gathered around my makeshift desk and listened intently to each exchange; the patient in question appeared entirely comfortable with this. I tried in vain to disperse the audience. I found myself whispering, as discreetly as possible, "When was the first day of your last menstrual period?" as the nurse tried to distract the women with more contraceptive demonstrations.

Then followed a whirlwind of Pap tests, by three practitioners in three exam rooms, with one interpreter dashing from room to room. By the end of the morning, we'd done six Pap tests, discovered a pelvic mass, diagnosed a pregnancy, and written four prescriptions for birth control.

It was a satisfying morning. I felt confident that the visit had solidified prior knowledge and would result in dissemination of new information to the Karen community. I anticipated that the women would feel more confident discussing women's health issues with health providers in the future, and that there would be increased screening uptake.

More than that, though, the group visit experience was unexpectedly moving. I was the guest: hearing stories of a jungle tree bark that would prevent pregnancy; watching the women banter with each other; answering their sometimes simple, sometimes sophisticated questions on pelvic anatomy. For once, I was the odd one out: they had the solidarity in numbers, language, culture. It was a reversal of positions. I felt equally humbled and privileged.

At the end of the morning, one of the women looped her arm through mine as we walked back to the waiting room. It wasn't just me, then, that felt that meeting in a group setting had done more for doctor-patient rapport than any private visit had.

"Thank you, teacher," she said in careful English.

I didn't let the interpreter correct her. She understood the role of physician perfectly.

17

As we reviewed the Karen women's health group visit after their departure, the medical student sighed, "They were adorable."

I'd run across this sentiment before, in all sort of contexts. "My constituents want their refugee families by Christmas!" I'd heard a mayor say about his small town's frustrations with delays in the private sponsorship system. "We are in love with our refugee family. Smitten!" wrote a blogger about the Iranian family for which her church was responsible.

I call this phenomenon maternalism—the misapplication of motherly sentiments that serve to infantilize the object of care. I first encountered this as a child, watching adults outside the family interact with my older sister, Julia, who has cerebral palsy. She pushed a little yellow walker, braced legs moving jerkily, and her speech was unclear. There was nothing wrong with her mind, though. I'd watch cashiers carefully enunciate their words, or ladies at church rummage in their purses for peppermints, and cringe. *She's not a baby!* I would think. *She's eight!* And later, *Eleven! Fourteen! Seventeen!* I can't say how it felt to be treated that way, but from my view, the sister on the sidelines, their concern diminished her; what she deserved was respect. My medical training emphasized avoiding paternalism, the use of physician authority to restrict the freedom and responsibilities of patients in their supposed best interest. But maternalism was never mentioned.

When I was a resident running the family practice ward, I would come up to the unit after supper to finish dictations and complete paperwork. At the end of the evening, I'd ask the charge nurse if there were any patients she was concerned about or orders that needed to be written. Having tied up all the loose ends, I'd head to the basement call room, where the resident on duty spent the night. I distinctly remember how I felt walking down the corridor at eleven at night. The ward was hushed and still, with the patients' lights off and just one or two staff at the nursing station. Heading back to the elevator, I walked past rooms of four beds apiece with patients resting under blue cotton blankets. I had brought my charges through another day.

Now, a few years later, I made the rounds of my own children every night before bed. The gratification as I adjusted the covers over small sleeping bodies was remarkably similar to walking down the corridor of 7B late at night—the sense of having tucked the kids in for the night. It was a powerful emotion, a combination of affection and respect for those under my care, the satisfaction of having managed the day's problems, the weight of responsibility, and humility and gratitude for my own position.

I raised New Zealand rabbits as a kid; they were white with ruby eyes. The smell of the nesting box with eight kits in it was strangely heady to a thirteen-year-old, offering the intimate smell of birth, fur, and urine, at the same time attractive and repulsive. The scent was the essence of something that I couldn't quite recognize.

As a mother, twenty years later, not many things moved me as strongly as lifting the lids from my Rubbermaid bins of newborn baby clothes, long since packed away. It was the smell that made me weak in the knees. It wasn't exactly a baby scent, and it wasn't even entirely pleasant. It was the smell of laundry detergent brands I had used back then, and the smell of the houses my babies were raised in. There was a musty scent, a whiff of spit-up, the faintest trace of Johnson's baby shampoo. I could hold a newborn onesie to my face, breathe it in, and feel dizzy with nostalgia. Pete did not have the same inclination to do this.

It took me years to connect the two scents. The smell of the rabbit nest was motherhood; the smell of the baby clothes was that of the nest I'd made for my own children. That it affected me so strongly made sense: I'd always loved to nurture things. Dolls, tadpoles, rabbits, sheep, a German Shepherd, petri dishes inoculated with E. coli—if it could grow, I wanted to be there cheering it on. At eight, I wanted to be a farmer; at eighteen, a veterinarian. At twenty-eight, I finished a family medicine residency. Now I spent my evenings puttering in the garden.

Nurturing is a natural fit with medicine. So are other

qualities commonly considered maternal: tenderness, warmth, the ability to comfort. What my patients at the refugee clinic needed most, though, was to regain independence. I saw the clinic as a temporary home, a safe and familiar place where patients could anchor themselves in their first year in the country. It was a kind of nest, and the goal was to launch them from it.

Sometimes I'd run into former patients years later.

"Two items?" asked the Winners change room attendant, briskly, with accented English. And then, seeing my face: "Bridge Clinic!" The clinic was just a memory, something she'd long since moved on from, and witnessing her settled in her new life brought me joy. Or was it maternal pride?

Maternalism risked infantilizing the patient just as paternalism did. I'd noticed that refugees seemed particularly able to inspire and amplify maternal feelings in medical practitioners, sponsors, and other front-line workers. I had a theory about that. Many refugees had child-like qualities: they had difficulty communicating in English, they were initially dependent on others, and they were deferential. These features made them non-threatening, and set up an automatic power differential. Helpers swooped in. Paternalism exerted power deliberately; I worried that maternalism did too, just more subtly.

I enjoyed my compliant patients, even as I urged them to self-advocate. In general, refugees were less demanding than the Canadian-born patients at my first practice in Kitsilano, although the trends varied by group. Patient behaviour appeared to be influenced by cultural attitudes toward doctors; the medical system with which patients were familiar; gender; education; and wealth and status prior to coming to

Canada. Most patients were grateful to finally have access to medical treatment, while others protested the Canadian wait times and claimed they'd received better care in the refugee camp.

I was guilty of checking the schedule of interpreters booked for my patients at the start of clinic and projecting, based on the languages listed, whether the day would unfold at a peaceful pace or progress at breakneck speed and end with me staying an hour late to catch up on paperwork. Ideally, there was a mix of patients, and those with higher needs were balanced by those who required less. My heart could sink or soar depending on the list.

Some groups were more medically complex than others. The Bhutanese patients had lived in refugee camps since the 1980s and their trauma history, if any, was remote. Other groups had fled recent conflict and their fresh wounds—physical and psychological—necessitated more intense care. Clinicians have finite reserves of time, patience, and resilience, and some patients tax these more than others. It's natural to prefer the less depleting patient encounters. I enjoy some patient visits more than others in the same way that I prefer my daughter lying in the hammock with a book for hours on end to my son thudding down the stairs in a cardboard box. At home and at the clinic, some days I want fewer demands and more compliance. Some days I want my own job made easier.

An attitude that I frequently encountered outside of the clinic was the expectation that refugees act from a position of obligation and inferiority. "We helped a refugee family, once; we let them stay in the suite over our garage for next to nothing," began a woman I'd just met at a birthday party, upon learning what I did for a living. I knew exactly what was coming next, because I'd heard a variation of it countless times before: "And they asked if our son could stop shooting hoops in the driveway after eight, because it kept the baby awake."

The other women gathered in the kitchen shook their heads at the gall, the lack of proper gratitude. Someone chimed in, "Our church helped out a Congolese family for an entire year, and then they left for a Pentecostal church." Sympathetic murmurs. "And! They didn't want to buy their clothes second-hand."

I once came across an article on assisting children with special needs, contrasting the helper to the helped.[1] Helping affirms capacity, worth, and superiority; being helped implies deficiency, burden, and inferiority. The helper is owed; the helped is obligated. Providing help, one's vulnerability is masked, while the other's is highlighted. Helping others is not necessarily altruistic.

The article made me examine my motivation for the work I did. Was I drawn to care for marginalized populations because of a moral imperative, or because the distinction between the capable helper and the deficient recipient was that much clearer? But gifts from patients made me uncomfortable precisely because I worried that the patient felt obligated to me. Much of my work focused on affirming the patient's own worth and capacity. I knew that my strongest quality as a physician was the ability to make patients feel they were being treated as equals.

When I prepared a presentation on refugee health for a group of private sponsors on Vancouver Island a few months later, I made the final slide about the contrast between helper and helped. I wondered whether it was unfair to challenge the motivation of well-meaning volunteers. I needn't have worried. It was the most well-received part of the presentation, prompting an audience-led discussion of how one might smooth the differences in position of sponsor and refugee. I was relieved. I wanted to encourage their generosity. I just wanted a little dose of self-reflection to accompany it.

18

WHEN OUR CLINIC DID A patient survey, several respondents noted favourably: *The doctor always asks about my house.* It was true. I did, although I had no idea that patients appreciated it so much. I asked because it was a benign entry into a patient visit, with easy questions to answer, and it yielded useful information. Five people in a three-bedroom, top-floor apartment overlooking New Westminster had completely different implications for health than the same family in a two-bedroom, windowless basement suite a mile and a half from the nearest bus stop.

"Tell me about your home," I'd say. "How many bedrooms? Who sleeps where? Is there a quiet place to study? Is it bright? Is it adequate?"

Some patients who moved up from cooking over fires in jungle camps to apartments in downtown Langley needed to be taught to operate a stove. They felt they lived like kings. Others gave up beautiful family estates with gardens in the Middle East for a dark, mouldy rental. They were reminded constantly of what they had lost.

Some cultural groups clustered together, while others scattered widely. Almost all my Bhutanese patients lived in one of two apartment complexes in Coquitlam. Iraqi patients tended to settle where they felt they were least likely to encounter other Iraqis.

The Haddads lived in a two-bedroom apartment in Surrey.

"How's your place?" I asked Yusef. "How are your neighbours?"

"No good," he said. "Brown people everywhere." He mimed a turban on his head.

I looked at the address on file. I had lived in the area years before. It had a sizable Punjabi Sikh population.

"I want to live with Canadians," Yusef went on earnestly.

"They are Canadians." I knew what he would say next, because I'd had this conversation with other patients.

"Canadians like you." He pointed at my face. "White."

"I'm not any more Canadian than your neighbours are," I said. "My parents were immigrants." Both of my parents had emigrated from the Netherlands as children.

That made no difference to him. "I want to live with white people," he said. "Not Surrey. Where?"

"All of Greater Vancouver is very multicultural," I told him. "Everyone's mixed together—Asians, Africans, Middle Easterners, Europeans." I loved the city's diversity. Pete and I were pleased that our kids' school had an ethnic mix that was representative of Vancouver, rather than the homogenous Dutch composition of our own childhood classrooms, comfortable though that had been. I'd assumed that refugees would feel more at home in a multicultural city than in one where they were the only visible minority.

"No good," he said again.

"You could try somewhere in the Interior," I said. "You might like Kelowna."

I was half joking. I was at a loss as to what to advise him. His stated preference for white neighbours was at odds with Canadian multiculturalism, but he'd only been in the country for three months. I couldn't pretend to understand the culture, history, and experiences that informed his mindset. While the conversation disturbed me, I didn't judge him for it. I wondered, though, if my lenience was a luxury I could afford because I was white.

It wasn't the first time I'd encountered prejudice at the clinic. Another patient, years before, appeared disgruntled the moment I called him from the waiting room. Unsmiling, he grabbed his coat and cane and walked toward us as aggressively as his limp would allow.

I introduced the medical student and asked his permission for her to join us. He gave a curt nod and charged past us, down the hall toward the exam room.

We followed behind, and I gestured to the student to observe his gait: he favoured his left leg, swinging it out to the side with each step so that his foot wouldn't strike the floor. He had sustained a spinal cord injury in a bomb blast in Iraq five years earlier.

He came straight to the point once he'd been seated. "You send me to Korean doctor!" he accused. I'd referred him to a neurologist. I found the report and looked at the letterhead.

"Dr. Nakamura is Japanese-Canadian," I said.

He waved his hand impatiently. "This," he said. He put an index finger next to each eye and pulled upward, his eyes slanted slits. He turned to the medical student and repeated the gesture, emphatically. The student was of Chinese descent.

"Send me to different doctor," said the patient. "Not that kind."

"The fact that Dr. Nakamura is Asian has nothing to do with his abilities as a doctor," I said. "I won't make a second referral based on that." He humphed with displeasure but didn't protest further. I went on to review the recommendations in the consult letter with him.

I wondered what to do about the slant-eye caricature. Perhaps it was just an effort at communication by someone with a language barrier. Maybe refusing the second referral was enough of a stand for today. He was a recent arrival, and immersion in Canadian culture would eventually teach him more tolerance, I reasoned. And so I left it.

The visit ended, and we saw the next patient, and the next, a steady stream through the afternoon. I meant to debrief with the student, but we were caught up in a whirlwind of paperwork at the day's end, and then she was gone. Her rotation was over, and we never discussed what happened in that exam room.

I began to wonder what was worse, his gesture or my allowing it. For months and then years, I watched for her at the clinic and at conferences. At first, I wanted to explain. Then, I wanted to ask forgiveness. I couldn't do either. I didn't find her.

My patients faced discrimination themselves, of course. A few months before, after we'd finished a morning of six consecutive Arabic-speaking patients, Hani had seemed preoccupied. "Is everything okay?" I'd asked.

"I'm upset about the shooting," she had confessed.

So was I. So was the entire nation. A few days before, a twenty-four-year-old Canadian soldier was killed while on sentry duty at the National War Memorial on Parliament Hill in Ottawa. He was shot twice in the back by a lone assailant. Passersby had rushed to perform CPR, and had said the Lord's Prayer with him as he lay dying on the grass.

The gunman, Michael Zehaf-Bibeau, had gone on to storm the Parliament buildings, where he died in a shootout. He was Muslim, and the shootings were deemed a terrorist act.

The soldier who died was Nathan Cirillo, and the pictures of him on the news, taken from his Facebook account, made the events all the more horrifying: kind eyes, a wide smile, his young son in the crook of his arm, his dogs in his lap.

Hani's eyes were filled with tears. "On SkyTrain now, I feel ashamed of my headscarf."

"Did anyone say anything to you?" I pressed.

Once one of my Afghani patients, a thirty-year-old father of two, had told me casually that he'd been called a terrorist on public transit. He was one of the Pashtun men who'd interpreted for the Canadian military during its mission there, and was offered refugee status in Canada for his own safety when the military pulled out in 2011. I'd been angrier than he was.

"No. No," Hani said quickly. "Nothing has happened. I just feel people looking at me."

I realized that I'd always had the luxury of being inconspicuous. When I take public transit, I enjoy the swaying masses that crowd the SkyTrain cars, a heterogeneous blur of shapes and colours, backpacks and strollers, beards and ponytails. I feel absorbed into the throng. I'd assumed everybody did.

I have never waited at a bus stop, shopped for groceries, or walked through a neighbourhood without the implicit understanding that I have every right to be there. My belonging is never in question. I am only a second-generation Canadian, but I cannot be told to return to a country a half-world away because my features and dress give no hint as to where that might be. It is a privilege I hadn't recognized I held.

I live where refugees are least likely to settle in Vancouver: on the North Shore. Due to the cost of living, refugees tend to migrate south and east from Vancouver proper to Richmond, Surrey, Burnaby, and Coquitlam.

For my first years in practice I lived in East Vancouver with my husband and young family. We were squeezed onto a twenty-five-foot-wide lot, in a one-hundred-year-old Edwardian house with a sleeping porch off the master bedroom, eaves pressed against our neighbour's. We turned thirty and the vibrancy of urban living lost its appeal. At night, our house throbbed with the neighbour's music, and a new nozzle on the garden hose would disappear within days.

We moved to Deep Cove, to a weathered house on stilts overlooking Indian Arm, screens of massive firs and cedars between us and the neighbours.

"It's so civilized!" I remarked to Pete shortly after we moved into the neighbourhood. Properties were kept uniformly tidy. It was safe enough that not only could we forgo a house alarm, we could leave the doors unlocked. No one rummaged through the blue bin on recycling day. We'd go to the Cineplex Esplanade or White Spot restaurant, and I'd look around at the homogeneous crowd around us and feel a camaraderie: we were all hard-working families who took the canoe out on weekends. And virtually everyone, I noticed as an afterthought, was white.

One day as I drove up Cove Cliff Road toward home, I saw a figure walking a mid-sized dog. I didn't recognize the dog, a blue merle Australian shepherd, and slowed as I approached what I assumed was a new neighbour. He wore brown dress pants and a cream shirt with the sleeves rolled up. I passed him and glanced at his face. He looked Iranian.

My unfiltered gut response, which horrified me even as I registered it, was *What is he doing here?* I instantly felt ashamed. Did I welcome immigrants, so long as they kept to my exam room and the suburbs east of Vancouver? Was working at a refugee clinic while living in an affluent North Shore community a farce? I tried to tease my response apart. Part of it was the surprise. A Persian man walking a dog in my neighbourhood was an undeniably unusual event. The other issue was that I associated Iranians with the clinic. Deep Cove, peaceful and calm, was where I sought respite from my work. The sighting felt like a jarring crossover of work life into my personal life.

When I met him walking in the woods a few days later, I introduced myself and welcomed him to the neighbourhood. His name was Saeed, he told me with a Farsi accent. He had just moved with his wife and two young sons into the house over the hill.

We have often crossed paths since, he with his dog or his sons on bikes, and I going for a run. We always stop to chat.

19

PULLED A CHART FROM THE rack at the front desk and read the name of the next walk-in patient. *Jesus.* I'd seen enough Colombian refugee claimants to know this one. "Hey-Soos?" I called confidently into the crowded waiting room. No one moved. "Hey-Soos?" I tried again. Two dozen faces gazed at me impassively. Then a Latino man politely raised his hand.

"I'm Jesus," he said, pronouncing it like an evangelical preacher. "I'm Jesus, if that's who you're looking for."

It frustrated me that the clinic expected physicians to retrieve their own patients from the waiting room and escort them to the exam room. For years, I had chafed at the inefficiency of this system. I wanted to revolve through two exam rooms, with the next patient always ready in the other room, seated by the medical office assistant. When the clinic commissioned a community engagement survey, the most interesting part was the unsolicited comments. One patient reminisced, "The doctor would personally call me by name from the waiting room. Years later, I feel warm inside remembering that." Other respondents also mentioned this practice fondly. All those years rushing down the hall to call the next patient, impatient to get to the real work, and I'd had no idea that this inconvenience to me was therapeutic for the patient.

I made a concerted effort to learn patients' names, with proper pronunciation. I would read the name on the chart and make a valiant attempt at it. *Ahdiyeh?* The patient would nod, but with just enough hesitation that I knew they were humouring me. "You say it," I'd say, and they would, quick and effortless. I'd try to mimic them, struggling with the foreign phonemes. Patients always looked one part delighted at my efforts and one part embarrassed for me. I felt a little foolish sometimes, but if I expected patients to push past their self-consciousness to practice English, rehearsing their names was the least I could do.

Sometimes the name on the chart wasn't recognizable to the patient. The Myanmar patients came from a culture where they could change their name at will, to reflect a change in life. They had no surnames, and their first names often incorporated an honorific title. A boy named Htay might grow up to be called Ko ("older brother") Htay, or Saw ("mister") Htay. For the purposes of Canadian immigration paperwork, though, one name had to be designated the surname. And so, addressing a patient with a chart labelled *Saw, Htay* as "Mr. Saw" or "Htay" or "Htay Saw" did not actually qualify as calling him by name. Although our clinic forbade writing on the chart cover, once I sleuthed the patient's true name, I pencilled it onto the chart label. I was certain that rapport was jeopardized by addressing patients by a name that was not theirs.

There were so many Abdullahs and Farzanahs coming through the clinic that it was hard to keep them straight. The endless spelling variants didn't help: Mohammed, Muhammad, and Mohamad were all my patients; so was Moh'd, his name apparently abbreviated on an application form on the other side of the world a year ago and now his immutable Canadian legal name. Husband, wife, and children—whether from Iraq, Bhutan, or Somalia—rarely shared a surname, making it challenging to determine and recall family relationships.

If I didn't have both the chart and the patient in front of me, I found it very difficult to match the history to the patient. In all my years at the clinic, I'd had one patient named Brian. I can still recall his face and detailed medical history, because his name was distinct and familiar.

There were other unforgettable names. Some of the Myanmar children relocating from a jungle camp in Thailand to downtown Langley were named for British rock stars. An optimistic new mother named her Canadian-born infant son Skilful, but misspelled it.

When I had been pregnant with my third child, a daughter, I had considered every female patient's name as a contender. My favourites were the Hispanic names: Luciana, Catalina, Alessandra. I cared more about the aesthetics of a name than its meaning. I knew my considerations were superficial when I noted the significance of names to my patients.

One of my Iranian families had fled to Canada when they converted from Islam to Christianity. On their second visit with me, the father drew some paperwork from his briefcase. "Name change for our son," he said, nodding at the four-year-old boy sitting on his wife's lap. "Please sign."

I looked over the documents. They were requesting a name change from Mohammed to Joshua.

In the end, I named my daughter Ariana, to mixed reviews at work. "That's the name of the Afghani airline," the Farsi interpreter informed me doubtfully.

"We plan to call her Aria, after my grandmother," I reassured her.

With increasing dismay, she replied, "But Aria's a Persian boy's name!"

20

THE FIRST TIME I SAW Li he was seated at the end of a pew in the waiting room, trembling. It wasn't a fine hand tremor or the bobbing head of the elderly, but a visible vibration of his entire body. His face had such a strange grey-white sheen to it that I wondered briefly if he was wearing makeup. I introduced myself and he clung to my hand with both of his, head tilted back, a gesture of supplication so archaic and desperate that I felt embarrassed. The Mandarin interpreter sat next to him, looking nonplussed and wearing a throat-closing amount of perfume.

In the exam room, the interpreter unhurriedly hung up her coat, retied her scarf, and settled back in her chair. "How are your children, Doctor? How old are they now?"

The patient sat on the edge of his seat, knees apart and legs angled back under the chair. Suddenly he leaned back, dug in the front pocket of his jeans, and handed me a business card:

THOMAS STRIKER
LAWYER – AVOCAT – ABOGADO
900 W GEORGIA STREET, VANCOUVER

"Lawyer sent him," said the interpreter. "Needs a letter."

It wasn't uncommon for immigration lawyers to direct asylum seekers to our clinic for a medical legal report to document injuries sustained during persecution in their country of origin. Li, I learned, had been held in a "re-education by labour" camp in China for two years for practising Falun Gong, a Chinese spiritual movement. During his imprisonment he'd been beaten with electric batons, and he had the scars to prove it, he told me. His wife had died in the camp.

I pulled out a ruler, marked to the millimetre, and seated him on the exam table. "I know it's painful to recall the awful things that happened to you in the past," I said, "but the more information you can provide, the more detailed the report I can write, and the better the case your lawyer can make." The interpreter relayed this, and Li nodded. "Let's go from head to toe," I said. "Tell me about any injuries, and show me any scars."

The Istanbul Protocol is a set of international guidelines for the documentation of torture and its consequences, adopted by the United Nations in 1999. At eighty-three pages, it had been my weekend reading a few months earlier. After a Saturday breakfast of pancakes and bacon, I'd sat on the couch with my coffee to read the chapter, "Beatings and Other Forms of Blunt Trauma." I'd done some yard work and then reluctantly read "Suspension" and "Other Positional Torture." Before we brought the kids to the pool I'd planned to read about asphyxiation, but I couldn't do it. The manual is a sickening read, and I regretted trying to work it into a Saturday with my family.

The Istanbul Protocol's "Annex III: Anatomical Drawings for Documentation of Torture and Ill-Treatment" is a set of printable blank diagrams of the human body on which to mark the patient's injuries. There are eight pages, viewing the body from every angle: front, rear, side. There are close-up diagrams of the genitals and the soles of the feet. An entire page is devoted to hands. There's a skeleton on which to document bony injuries, and thirty-two teeth sketched in grim, forensic detail. I printed the package while Li changed into a gown.

He began by pointing to a scar on his chest, a pale area the size of a credit card.

"Electric baton," said the interpreter. "During interrogation."

I measured it out with my ruler, then carefully shaded in a rectangular area on the chest of the figure on my printout, drew an arrow to it, and labelled it, "Depigmented patch, irregular margins, 8.3 cm wide × 5.5 cm high."

For the next thirty minutes I measured and described Li's scars as precisely as I could, and he told me the circumstances of each injury. At the end, the figure on my page had markings on almost every surface of its body and the patient retched into the sink.

I told him I was sorry we'd had to do this. I told him I was sorry that he'd suffered so much, and that he didn't deserve any of it. I told him that I'd like to see him again in two weeks, and that I'd connect with his lawyer in the meantime.

When I saw Li next he leapt to his feet when I walked into the waiting room. He was as shaky and pale as the first visit, but managed a smile. The clinic had been unable to book a Mandarin interpreter, so once in the exam room I dialed the Provincial Language Service. We were soon connected to an interpreter who, from the sounds of it, was going through the grocery store checkout with kids in tow. I put her on speakerphone and positioned the phone on the counter, midway between me and the patient.

Li leaned toward it and started talking immediately, urgently.

"He says that last time he didn't tell you everything that happened," said the interpreter. "He says some things happened that didn't leave scars that you can see."

Li spoke so forcefully that the interpreter struggled to get him to pause, so she could relay the story to me, piece by piece. The patient had been sexually assaulted by the prison guards, on multiple occasions. He described the first attack in awful detail, and then moved on to the second.

The interpreter balked. "I won't continue," she said suddenly.

"Pardon me?" I said. Li paused, mid-story, confused.

"I'm going to hang up."

"But we're not finished!"

"I have children, you know!" She sounded like she was about to cry. "I won't be able to sleep at night." She was still in the store; I could hear the beep of scanners.

I couldn't believe it. How could she complain about having to hear these stories when the patient had had to experience them? It was her job to translate whatever the patient disclosed, not to fold when the topic got uncomfortable. I had children, too, and I was already having trouble sleeping at night from countless stories like this one, but I was soldiering on. I was angry that she sought self-preservation, and I was angry that it was too late for me.

"Don't hang up," I said. "We won't talk anymore about what happened to him. We'll move on to asking about his mood and sleep."

I spent the next Saturday morning composing the medical legal report, as I'd written dozens of others over the years. I outlined my credentials, stated the trauma history provided by the patient, detailed the physical injuries, and commented on any psychological distress. I described Li's scars in painstaking detail and emailed a draft report to the lawyer.

Thomas Striker responded on Monday morning. "Could you state definitively that the scars were sustained from beatings with electric batons?" he asked.

I couldn't. The scars were non-specific. Electrical burns typically produced one to three millimetre reddish brown circular lesions, according to the Istanbul Protocol, and Li's scars did not fit this description.

The lawyer responded with a gruesome image of a disfigured face covered with crusted, blackened areas of skin. "Sorry!" he wrote. "But I Googled 'electric baton injuries' and discovered this. It doesn't resemble the red dots you said were typical. Perhaps such injuries can have a different appearance than what's described in the Istanbul Protocol?"

The image appeared to show an acute injury, not scarring, I replied. I was happy to cite a medical source that described alternate scarring patterns from electrocution injury, but I wasn't aware of any beyond the Istanbul Protocol. Google Images didn't count.

"Sorry to be a pest," Thomas's next email began. He pushed for stronger wording in my report. I knew he was simply doing his job. But so was I, and I wouldn't budge. I was limited to the findings from a physical exam and the evidence in the medical literature. I might be the patient's advocate, but no matter how strongly I might want Li to win his case, I wasn't the adjudicator.

Li began every visit by recounting the story of the first time he was sexually assaulted in the camp.

"He already told us this," the interpreter said to me during the third or fourth retelling.

It felt heartless to interrupt, but it wasn't the best use of our visits, either. I reminded him that we'd documented his experiences in the medical legal report for his hearing. I acknowledged that terrible things had happened to him. I assured him that I'd put in a referral to VAST for counselling. I redirected him to his current day-to-day life.

"How's your sleep, Li?"

"Awake all night, every night. Only sleep during day."

"What do you do at night?" I guessed that he was on the Internet, a common preoccupation among my traumatized patients.

I was wrong. He sat in a chair from sunset to sunrise, facing the door, waiting for something to happen to him. He described how the night before, he wanted to pull the blinds against the harsh glow of the streetlights. Convinced that there were snipers outside, he had to screw up his courage and sidle up to the window, hugging the wall, and quickly yank down the shades before diving for the floor.

Li had other symptoms of post-traumatic stress disorder, such as nightmares and fearful avoidance of men in uniform, and I started him on sertraline. With counselling, medication, and support from his lawyer and me, he slowly improved over the next months. He was extremely grateful for this.

"For everything Canada has done for me, I wish to donate my corneas," he began one visit.

I was caught by surprise. This was a complete departure from our usual conversation, which centred on his mental health and upcoming legal hearing.

"Please arrange this!" he pressed.

I knew little about organ and tissue donation, beyond signing up when one got a driver's license. "Let's wait for the results of your hearing," I suggested. "If your refugee claim is successful, I'll get the information on cornea donation for you."

"I don't want to wait! Even if I go back to China, I wish to donate my corneas to Canadian children," he continued, through the interpreter. "How would I arrange to transport my corneas back to Canada?"

Suddenly I had an unsettling thought. Surely he wasn't suggesting that he donate his corneas now, while he was alive? The strange nature of his request and his insistence on following it through raised red flags for me. I wondered if this were a psychotic feature related to his PTSD. China had been accused of trafficking organs harvested from Falun Gong practitioners. Perhaps his trauma history was related to this request.

"I wish to donate them to blind children!" he said urgently. "I am so grateful to Canada for everyone's kindness. It is the only thing I can think of to give back."

I had to clarify, and I couldn't think of an indirect way to do so. "Li," I said carefully. "Do you mean that you wish to donate your corneas now? Or after your death?"

He and the interpreter stared at me, and there was an incredulous pause. Li looked so perturbed by my question that I felt embarrassed that I'd asked it. "When I'm dead, of course!"

He won his claim. He obtained a work permit and provincial health insurance. His PTSD symptoms faded rapidly. I arranged to transfer him to a community family physician. He never brought up cornea donation again.

21

"THEY TOOK EVERYTHING ELSE FROM me," Junah told me one afternoon in February. "My son, my home, my country. The only thing they couldn't take was my religion." It was her one comfort. I asked if she believed in life after this one. She did. "Imagine meeting the one who created you," she marvelled. "He'll ask if you believed faithfully, and he will judge." Implicit in her faith was the conviction that those who had wronged her family would face divine justice.

The Haddads were Muslim, but they didn't attend a mosque. They avoided places where other Iraqis might congregate. They were intent on embracing Canadian life; in shaking off their past, their attachment to religious customs loosened as well. They prayed, though, and observed Ramadan.

I routinely ask patients about religion. It is relevant to health in many ways: Muslims may fast during Ramadan; the Baha'í are typically vegetarian; Christians are less likely to terminate an unplanned pregnancy. Religion can offer community and a framework to understand suffering. I was cautious about how I asked, aware that many of my patients became refugees after someone in authority enquired about their religion.

I had increasing numbers of patients from Iraq, Iran, and Syria, and I wanted to brush up on my knowledge of the history of the Middle East. It became my bedtime reading. I was reading up on Saddam Hussein one night when I came across a video, footage of the purge of the Ba'ath Party in 1968, narrated by Christopher Hitchens. A young Saddam lounged on the stage, puffing casually on a cigar, as terrified party members were escorted out of the assembly to their executions. I thought of Junah's steadfast belief in justice in the next life, and I understood her position. How could that kind of evil go unpunished?

That night I dreamed that I was caught in crossfire in Baghdad. I woke before dawn, exhausted. I wasn't consciously preoccupied with my patients' stories of trauma outside of clinic hours, but my dreams hadn't been peaceful for years. I had nightmares of torture, fleeing my home, being sent to a work camp. When the scenes weren't directly lifted from patient stories, they still revolved around death: finding my cat's lifeless body, my son drowning, a co-worker being assassinated. The images were second-hand, I protested, frustrated when they would cling to me for hours after waking. They were just faint impressions of what the actual horror must have been like for my patients. They were only dreams.

Junah's comments about judgement in the afterlife prompted me to revisit my own beliefs on the subject. I delved into the history, theology, and literature around the Christian concept of hell. I resisted the idea of eternal conscious torment for unbelievers. But how could an afterlife without punishment be just? It was fascinating but unsettling study. Part of me thought that devoting so many hours of this life to contemplating the details of a possible next existence couldn't be right.

Driving into town with my six-year-old to run errands on a Saturday afternoon in May, I was distracted from my ruminations about divine judgement by the never-ending stream of tangential questions from the back seat. "Why do Chinese people use Chinese writing?" Leif asked as we passed through Vancouver's Chinatown. "Why would they use something so hard?"

Suddenly I had a question of my own. "Leif, do you know what hell is?"

"No! What is it?" he asked with interest. I was amazed. And relieved. I pointed out a giant neon rickshaw sign to divert him from pressing for an answer.

Later that night I emailed my sisters: "How old were you when you learned what hell was?"

One was five, one couldn't remember, one didn't reply. "How about you?" asked the one who couldn't remember.

"Six months," I said. Not really. But it was before I could swim, or ride a bike. Four, I think.

My childhood revolved around the New Westminster Christian Reformed Church. Grandparents, classmates, and neighbours were all part of the same Dutch immigrant community. John Knox Christian School was directly across the street from the church, on 13th Avenue. We lived three blocks away, my grandparents four. On Saturdays, my younger sister and I rode our bikes through the back alleys of north Burnaby with our school friends, collecting walnuts and exploring vacant lots. The next morning, we'd rejoin those same friends at church. I was wrapped in layers of community, snug and safe. I would recreate this community for my own children, if I could bring it back.

When I was six, my parents gave us Psalter Hymnals for Sinterklaas, the Dutch gift-giving celebration on December 5. A few years later we memorized the Heidelberg Catechism from the back of the book. It began: "What is your only comfort in life and in death?" I rattled off the answer, no pauses for the commas: "That I am not my own but belong body and soul both in life and in death to my faithful Saviour Jesus Christ." Every Sunday night we'd recite a portion to my parents and be rewarded with a sticker.

As a child, I loved the Christian Reformed community. I was more ambivalent about God Himself. I had a clear picture of Him in my mind: Caucasian, short and stocky, clean-shaven with black wavy hair, slumped on a throne with his chin in his right hand. It took me decades to sort out where this image came from. It was not my Dad, or the minister. It was an image of King Saul from our children's Bible, in one of his depressed states, listening to David the shepherd play his harp. You couldn't ever be sure if the king would be kindly or throw a spear at you in a rage. I'd known since preschool which one I deserved.

Now, as an adult, I attend St. John's Vancouver Anglican Church. The service offers excellent teaching, a connected parish community, and rich historical liturgy. The Book of Common Prayer has a prayer for physicians, that they might be granted "wisdom and skill, sympathy and patience" to "cheer, heal and sanctify the sick." I think it is remarkable that a liturgical book so neatly encapsulates the biopsychosocial-spiritual model of medicine that was taught with such effort when I started my training.

Sunday mornings were my respite, providing an opportunity for reflection and orientation that grounded me for another week at the refugee clinic. I had moved away from the focus on doctrinal details that characterized my upbringing. I cared about redemption and its practical application. I deeply admired the Jesuits, who combined priesthood with careers such as medicine or education. An article I read about Pope Francis, who is a Jesuit, described him as the rare combination of intellectual, practical, and humble. This was exactly the triad that described all my heroes, and that I strove to apply to my practice of both religion and medicine.

And so my preoccupation with the doctrine of hell that Junah's comments had prompted was out of character for me. It wasn't the only aspect of my spirituality that I struggled with. It seemed clear that God couldn't be trusted for personal safety. When my four-year-old was afraid in the night and I was about to reassure her of God's constant nearness and protection, just as I'd been comforted as a child, I hesitated, thinking of patients who'd depended on that same protection with disastrous results. I analyzed the hymns we sang in church. References to troubles and trusting seemed absurd when I considered the songs were mostly written by Englishmen during times of peace. When the Old Testament story of God ordering the slaughter of the babies of a newly conquered city was explained in a sermon, the theological justification angered me. Violence toward children wasn't the abstraction it had been for me a decade ago. My patients' experiences became the standard by which I measured everything. If a Christian concept couldn't be applied to someone who had been raped, been tortured, or watched their children die, I rejected it.

It wasn't until a psychologist joined our clinic that I learned that years of empathizing with stories of trauma can result in a disruption of the physician's own spirituality. Questioning one's frame of reference is a hallmark of vicarious traumatization, the psychological response of those who work with victims of trauma. It wasn't unusual for someone in my situation to struggle with despair and hopelessness.

At a staff meeting, we were offered suggestions to keep well: balance our personal and professional lives; offset a clinical caseload with other replenishing professional involvements; engage in political work for social change; seek out activities that provided hope and optimism. In short: medicine couldn't be all we did. We knew that. It was why none of the physicians at the clinic worked full-time. We knew we wouldn't last.

When my children were baptized, the prayer that the minister said afterward contained a line that perfectly captured how I wished to raise them: "Give them an inquiring and discerning heart, the courage and will to persevere, a spirit to know and love you, and the gift of joy and wonder in all your works."

I wanted those qualities, too. The first and last had always come easy for me. I worked at the third. It was the second that had become a challenge: *the courage and will to persevere.*

22

I WAS FOUR MONTHS PREGNANT AND barely managing to conceal it at work. It was June, and I no longer had the option of disguising my midsection with belted cardigans or careful layering. On discovering I had conceived, two months after our loss in December, I had been overwhelmed by the sense that this was grand work, this close involvement with birth, and, briefly, all else looked anemic. What else had the power of that immediate, unmistakable second pink line on the test strip laid on the bathroom counter? It stood for possibility, for the hope of a healthy pregnancy and a perfect newborn and another loved child. One slim line released a cascade of happy plans.

Pete and I were thrilled that I was pregnant again, at least as much as I could recall with our other three children. It didn't feel commonplace; my previous experiences—good and bad—made it that much more meaningful. It had been almost five years since Ariana was born. This me, the thirty-six-year-old mother of three, physician to refugees, living in Deep Cove, had never been pregnant. And yet, personal and professional experience with pregnancy loss had primed me to assume nothing. *I'm expecting* struck me as presumptuous. And so I was not expecting. I was simply pregnant.

As a resident, with no firsthand experience of pregnancy or parenting, I'd felt like an imposter when I tried to advise or reassure women. Now, after three kids, five pregnancies, and nine years of providing prenatal care, caring for mothers was one of my favourite aspects of my job. I was sympathetic to morning sickness, knew the pain of miscarriage, and never tired of finding the first fetal heartbeat. Still, I wasn't the expert.

"You are pregnant," I told my ten o'clock patient, a Somali woman dressed in vivid blocks of colours, with a long turquoise cloak over lemon-coloured pants. I was wearing my usual navy trousers, navy pumps, and a loose white blouse. Today my wardrobe didn't feel professional. It felt dull.

"No," she said, bright teeth flashing as she shook her head.

"The nurse checked your urine," I said. "The pregnancy test is positive."

Hani relayed this. The patient looked amused and said with the same certainty, "No."

"Your last menstrual period was six or eight weeks ago," I said, "and you're not using anything for family planning. Is that correct?"

She confirmed this. "But she knows she is not pregnant," said Hani. "She knows this."

"I would like to book you into the prenatal clinic," I said, "and do some blood tests."

Hani conferred with the patient. "She is not pregnant, but she will do those things if it will make you happy."

I saw her four weeks later. I thought urinary frequency or breast tenderness or morning sickness might have swayed her. She denied them all. I repeated the pregnancy test. A second pink line immediately showed up on the strip; I was annoyed with myself for allowing her certainty to inject doubt into the diagnosis.

She smiled as I tried to find a fetal heartbeat for the baby she knew didn't exist. Her dates weren't exact; she might be only ten weeks pregnant, or she might be twelve, when the fetal heart was typically audible by Doptone. There was no fetal heart. Most patients needed reassurance in this situation, but she simply pulled up the waistband of her pink and orange skirt and slipped on her shoes. I ordered an ultrasound.

The results came back a week later: *CRL 16 mm. No cardiac activity. Missed abortion.*

Crown rump length measures the distance from the top of the fetal head to the bum. Legs aren't included because they aren't present in very early pregnancy, and once they've formed, they are typically flexed. A result of 16 mm CRL correlates with an age of eight weeks. By the patient's menstrual dates, the fetus should have been at least two weeks further along in development.

I called the patient in.

"I had my period this morning," she said. "A heavy one."

I tried to explain that the baby had died a few weeks ago, and this was a miscarriage. I was ready to offer support and sympathy, but she didn't need any.

"I kept telling you," she said patiently. "I wasn't pregnant."

Technically, I'd met the standard of care. I couldn't think how any other medical course of action could have been justified. And yet, I felt that it was she who had graciously accommodated me. I had made Western medicine look a little ridiculous to both of us.

I was often reminded that I valued the medical component of clinic visits more highly than the patient did. Junah came to see me often, usually regarding paperwork for Layth, sometimes about headaches or fatigue. I didn't feel that I offered much as her doctor, but I did make her laugh at every visit. When she told me that just seeing my face lifted her spirits, I told her that there was no need for her to come into the exam room, then; I could just hurry by the waiting room, glance at her sitting there, and she could go home. She was delighted by this, either at the joke itself or the fact that a physician would be playful with her.

But Junah did not show up for that morning's appointment. After lunch I saw her in the waiting room, sitting with Hani. She looked upset. I joined them on the pew.

"She took the bus by herself for the first time," Hani explained, "but she didn't know which stop to get off at. So she just rode the bus up and down Broadway. Then she saw me walking back from lunch! She got off the bus and threw her arms around me, crying."

Navigation was often an issue for patients. Many were unfamiliar with street maps, and map reading was not as intuitive for them as it felt to someone who had been introduced to it in kindergarten. A Nigerian patient told me once, "I understand maps of Africa, with all the countries in different colours, but I'd never seen a city map with lines for roads."

Due to Vancouver's high cost of living, most patients resided in the suburbs, and public transportation to the clinic required multiple connections. Most patients couldn't read English. I'd overheard the Burmese interpreter giving directions to one of my patients: "Get off SkyTrain at King George Station. That's the one that starts with the letter that looks like this," sketching the three strokes of the letter K in the air with her forefinger. I was amazed that patients found us at all.

I ushered Junah and Hani into my exam room. "What can I help you with today?"

"Pregnancy test," said Hani, as Junah tried unsuccessfully not to look jubilant.

It had been eight months since she had told me she wished to conceive. She'd done the bloodwork and taken folic acid supplements. The wait list to see Medical Genetics was one year. She'd refused to hold off until then, and I didn't blame her. I guessed that no matter what a geneticist advised, Junah would pursue pregnancy.

"What was the first day of your last menstrual period?" I asked.

"It should have been three weeks ago, but it didn't come. The last one was May 2."

I took an orange-topped urine specimen container from the cupboard and wrote her initials on the label with a Sharpie. "Follow me to the bathroom," I said. "Fill the container one third full, put the lid on tightly, and leave it in the cupboard next to the sink."

The back of the cupboard opened onto the specimen room next door, where I waited. I heard the rustling of undress, a pause while she peed, a flush, the plunk of the specimen container being set on the metal shelf, and a click as the cupboard door swung shut. I opened my door to the cupboard and carefully removed the container. It was full to the brim and intimately warm. Like virtually all urine specimens I collected, the lid was set carefully on top but not screwed onto the container—a pending splash.

I tore open a pregnancy test package and used the soft plastic dropper to add two drops of Junah's urine to the sample well. I watched as the edge of urine wicked up the test strip, toward the pink stripe. I knew that in Room 146, Junah was praying silently and fervently. Kurt Vonnegut would say she was angling to change the shape of her story, to end things with an upswing, toward good fortune. As her physician, I was alert for potential dangers, and already I could imagine a half dozen that pregnancy could bring.

The urine washed over the test area, immediately producing a second solid pink line. I dropped the test into the trash, one of a dozen tests done that day, disposable slips of news of heartache and relief, joy and dismay, and went to give Junah the results.

"You're pregnant," I said. "Congratulations!" I meant it.

"*Alhamdulillah*," she said simply. Her prayers had been answered.

I pulled my pregnancy dating wheel from the drawer and matched up the dates. "You are seven weeks pregnant," I said. "Your due date is February 6."

I saw her again four weeks later. Every Tuesday afternoon for eight years the nurse and I had run a prenatal clinic for our refugee patients. All our patients, regardless of whether they were an Iraqi psychiatrist or a Somali villager, had the same basic concerns as all Canadians: the baby's health, their own physical symptoms, and financial resources. Every patient had the same smile spread across their face when I first ran the gelled Doppler probe over the uterus and picked up the steady, rapid drumming of a fetal heart, like hoof beats.

Junah was no different. We listened for a full holy minute, for one hundred forty-two tiny thuds. It was just Junah, Hani, and me; no one said a word. Pregnancy had not lost its power to amaze me. Regular clinical visits were almost always about a problem; the excitement of a pregnancy was a welcome change.

"It sounds good," I said finally, wiping the gel from her belly with a tissue.

Junah tugged her dress down over her belly and sat up. "If the baby is a boy, we will name him Ahmed," she said.

"Ahmed," I said. "I like that."

"If it is a girl, we will name her after you."

I was touched, and taken aback. "Thank you!" I said. "I'm honoured!" I loved the idea of a little Iraqi-Canadian girl named Martina being raised somewhere in Surrey.

Junah looked at me expectantly. I wasn't sure what she was waiting for.

"So?" she prompted, finally. "What is your name?"

"Oh! Martina." Although I'd introduced myself at our first meeting, she'd never addressed me by my first or even last name. I was simply *Doctor*.

"Martina," she said, carefully. It sounded different with an Arabic accent. It sounded perfect.

Junah slid off the exam table and settled in the chair. "As a woman, how do you be strong, but kind and loving and forgiving at the same time?" she asked me through the interpreter.

I knew that the joy of this pregnancy wouldn't cancel out her grief. I knew that having a child after the loss of another one was psychologically complex. She looked at me expectantly; she wanted an answer. And I recognized that this was less a patient asking a question of her doctor, and more a woman asking a question of another woman. I was moved that she would think I had any advice to give her. I knew that my life had not required the strength and forgiveness that hers had asked of her.

As I offered my thoughts, I wondered whether the twenty-five-year-old me would have had anything to say. I doubted it. In fact, I seriously doubted that anyone would have asked my fresh-faced self such a question in residency or early practice.

I'd always looked young, and had received countless remarks about it as a medical student. The comments were made in a marvelling or appreciative way, but as a novice struggling to project confidence and professionalism I didn't find them helpful.

Looking young became much more tolerable a few years later when I was twenty-eight and being taken for twenty-two. And then I had three children, and I'd been in practice a few years, and comments on my age trailed off. One day a patient said to me, "You must be about my age—from 1974?" I was shocked that he had nailed it. Shortly after, for the first time ever, I asked my hairdresser for a cut that would take a few years off. She gave me bangs.

It was a rare moment when I acknowledged that there might be advantages to not being or looking twenty-two. If my aging suggested to patients that I had lived even a little, and had learned something from it, I was grateful for it.

Grief is not weakness, I told Junah. Strength is compatible with tenderness. She could mourn Sami's death and honour his memory while living purposefully to care for Layth, Nadia, and the new baby. Junah listened intently to my responses. Little did she know that I absorbed her words about faith and optimism with a similar keen interest. Why was I so cautious and fearful about my own pregnancy when Junah embraced hers, serene despite intimate knowledge of the blows life could deal?

If she was expecting, I decided, then so was I.

23

I HAD A MORNING OF PEDIATRIC assessments, with patients ranging from an infant to sixteen-year-old Layth. The father of my first patient told me proudly how he'd weaned his three-year-old son since his last visit with me: "I showed him a picture of a gorilla nursing her baby and I told him, 'If you keep this up, this is what your mom will turn into.'"

Before I could comment, he went on: "I heard that in Canada, parents bring their kids to the zoo before the kids are old enough to go by themselves. Is that true?"

"Yes." Every North American zoo I'd ever visited had been packed with strollers, and I'd never thought to question whether it was appropriate.

He considered this, impressed. "In Canada, parents serve their kids," he observed. "Where I come from, kids serve their parents."

I found this commentary interesting, but I also had a developmental checklist to get through. I scanned for the questions that were relevant. Bike helmets and car seat safety were not; the family lived in a tiny apartment and relied on public transit.

"Can Johro use a sentence with five or more words?" I asked, trying to steer the conversation back to his son's assessment.

"Yes," said the father. And then, chattily, "When I take him to the park, I've noticed that parents here don't beat their children."

The visit ended with me briefing him on the legalities of corporal punishment in Canada. The breadth of what fell under the auspices of family medicine seemed to increase daily. I did not question, though, whether the discussion was necessary.

When I returned to the waiting room, Layth was standing with his arms folded over his chest, staring at the door he knew I'd come through, waiting impatiently to be called. When he saw me, he grabbed the yellow backpack at his feet and charged for the exam room. Yusef and Hani followed unhurriedly.

"He's annoyed that he's missing class for a doctor's appointment," Hani told me as we headed down the hall. I considered this excellent news.

"Tell me about school!" I prompted Layth, once we were settled in the exam room.

"I like it." He had been attending Grade 10 at the public high school two blocks from his home, with a modified course schedule and an aide, for the past seven months.

Yusef pulled his phone from his pocket, swiped and tapped, and passed it to me. It was a video clip of what appeared to be a high school musical production of *Charlie and the Chocolate*

Factory. "I didn't understand it," he said, pointing out Layth in an Oompa Loompa costume, "but I loved it."

Since my initial assessment, Layth had had a head CT, followed by an MRI for further detail. The report described the brain structures in crisp detail: *Thin corpus callosum. Decreased volume of cerebral white matter. Sulcal enlargement.*

The abnormalities didn't point definitively to a diagnosis. The images might be clear, exposing the anatomy of the brain in wondrous black and white detail, but the findings were nonspecific. Layth's condition remained a mystery. The pediatrician wrote in her consult letter that she agreed that he likely had a genetic syndrome, one rare enough that she didn't recognize it. Other than treatment for his chronic constipation, she had little to offer. The wait for Medical Genetics was over a year long.

Medicine might have come up short, but his teachers and classmates had transformed Layth's life. He was the calmest and most content he'd ever been, Yusef reported. He worked well with his aide, played soccer, and was learning English more quickly than his parents. The only concern was that some of his new vocabulary dismayed his parents with its vulgar bent. And he had started smoking cigarettes with his new friends.

Layth wasn't my first patient with a disability to thrive in Canada. A visually impaired Iranian man was guided into the office at his first visit by his two little daughters, each one holding a hand. He'd never seen either of their faces.

He played goalball, a Paralympic sport similar to indoor soccer, for the visually impaired. The ball had bells inside, the lines were cords taped to the floor and the goal was nine metres wide. Spectators had to maintain complete silence so that the players could hear the ball. When he first described the sport, I wondered if he was teasing me.

Within weeks of arrival in Canada, he was learning Braille for the first time and attending ESL classes. The lessons weren't coordinated, though. He described spelling out English words in Braille whose meaning he didn't yet know. In English class, he could hear the words but could not read the board or handouts. I was dismayed at the impracticality of this, but he laughed. He could only see opportunity.

Filling out a form regarding his disability one afternoon, I paused when I arrived at the question, *Does the patient require an assistive animal?* He was Muslim, and I was confident that he would want nothing to do with a dog. My policy was not to make assumptions, though, but to let the patient decide. I described the concept of a seeing-eye dog to the patient and his wife. Initially confused, huge smiles spread over their faces when they realized what I was suggesting.

"Doctor," interrupted his wife incredulously, "you are saying he could have a dog, attached to a rope, leading him around the city?" When I affirmed that this was, in essence, the idea, they laughed so hard that I blushed.

"Thank you," he finally gasped. "But no."

It was difficult for some patients to suddenly be presented with a solution to a chronic condition. An Afghani woman, deaf from birth and using a self-styled sign language with her family, learned from the ear, nose, and throat specialist that she was a candidate for a cochlear implant. She refused it, to her family's dismay. Her husband and teen daughter brought her to see me, hoping I could convince her to pursue the treatment.

The visit quickly erupted into shouting. "What if it makes

my migraines worse? What if I'm dizzy?" signed the patient, flicking her hair back angrily.

"You're so selfish!" shouted her husband, his hands signing furiously.

"You only think of yourself!" yelled the daughter. Then, just as I was about to rein them in, she pleaded: "We just want to hear your voice!"

Not everyone's life improved in the new country. "She was fine collecting firewood at the camp," one patient told me about his wife. "No one bothered us. Life is too complicated for her here."

His wife had an IQ of 70. When they left the refugee camp in Nepal for an apartment in Surrey, she struggled with simple tasks, such as using the stove and unlocking the front door. There were questions about her ability to care for her children.

"She was better off in the jungle," he said.

I silently agreed. It seemed a foregone conclusion that refugees with disabilities would benefit greatly from the Canadian system. Most did. We offered universal healthcare, world-class medical treatment, inclusive public education, and disability benefits. But not every patient viewed their condition as an impairment that needed to be corrected or supported. Some simply wanted to live as they were, in peace.

24

"PLEASE TAKE OFF ALL YOUR clothes," I said, miming the removal of my own shirt and pants, "and put on this gown." It was Tuesday afternoon, prenatal clinic, and the schedule was fully booked with a diverse set of patients. The first, a twenty-two-year-old Eritrean woman, was here for her physical exam.

The Tigrinya interpreter repeated my instructions, the patient smiled and nodded, and I pulled the soft blue curtain between us. I heard brief rustling; then all was still. I looked around the curtain to see her lying on the table, fully clothed.

"Please remove all your clothes," I reiterated, again supplementing with gestures. "I need you to take off your pants, shirt, bra, and underwear. Everything." She made an exclamation of understanding, and I turned back to my desk to prepare the requisitions.

When I next pulled back the curtain, the patient was lying full-length on the table, pants on, sweater half over her head, with her bra bunched around her throat. This time I addressed the interpreter directly. "She didn't understand. She's still dressed. All of her clothes must come off."

Shortly thereafter I heard a burst of activity behind the curtain. I looked in to see the patient standing on the table. My six-foot, pregnant patient was briskly disrobing while standing on a slender vinyl-covered exam table forty inches above the floor. I decided it was safer not to intervene and went back to assembling the speculum and swabs. A moment later she called out that she was ready.

And she was—lying on the table naked with the gown rolled up into a ball and tucked beneath her head.

The next patient, a Myanmar woman, was in for her first prenatal visit. This was her seventh pregnancy. I teased apart her obstetrical history through the interpreter. Two children were stillborn. It felt unholy to document the details in columns on a standardized form, but she held steady, and it seemed to her to be a matter of fact. My medical textbooks referred to *catastrophic obstetrical events*. *Catastrophe* comes from the Greek, *sudden turn*—a reversal of what is expected. It was my job to be vigilant, scanning the horizon for anything foreboding. I wanted the patient to enjoy this pregnancy, oblivious to threats.

Initial screening at the clinic had picked up microcytic anemia in her and her husband; further testing confirmed thalassemia trait in both. They were asymptomatic carriers. The only concern was that a future child might inherit the faulty gene from both parents, causing significant disease. I gave the clearest explanation I could, but the interpreter was confused, struggling for the Karen words, and my message appeared in the end to be relayed simply as, *You have bad blood.*

Weeks ago this woman had been living in a camp on the Thai-Myanmar border; now I was directing her to a geneticist, via a complicated bus route from her Langley apartment, for a condition she'd lived with for her entire life. I asked for questions, for her thoughts on my recommended plan, and she said simply, "Yes, Doctor."

The 2:30 patient needed to be offered prenatal genetic screening. Although this meant a complex discussion, I presented the same options to all patients, regardless of literacy level, ethnic origin, or religious practice. I'd been surprised too many times by patients' choices to feel comfortable making assumptions about their values.

I turned to my computer, typed "Down syndrome" into the Google search bar and clicked "Images." I turned the screen toward the patient, and she gazed at the gallery of faces, all with up-slanted eyes. Like every patient, no matter the country of origin, she nodded in recognition. The incidence of Trisomy 21 is just over one in a thousand births worldwide and affects all ethnicities.

She spoke in Swahili. "Mongolism," said the interpreter. "A man in her village looked like that."

"This is one of the conditions that the extra tests can diagnose," I told her.

I pulled a laminated chart from my drawer and explained that the likelihood of having a baby with Down syndrome increases with age. She was thirty years old, and her risk was about 1 in 840. It rises to 1 in 356 for a thirty-five-year-old, and shoots to 1 in 94 when a woman passes forty.[1]

I could see that she was lost in the numbers. "The blood test can give a more accurate prediction than this chart," I explained. "If it shows a very high risk, you could have further testing to say for certain whether the baby has the condition. That would involve putting a needle into your belly to get a sample of the fluid around the baby."

She looked alarmed at this. "She didn't do any tests with her other babies and they were healthy," said the interpreter. "Why does she need it with this one? Is there a problem, Doctor?" They both looked at me anxiously. She'd had no prenatal care for her other pregnancies; all were birthed successfully in her village hut with a midwife. Why was I complicating things?

"I have no reason to believe that your baby isn't healthy," I said. "It's your choice whether to have the extra testing."

This didn't reassure her. "You're the doctor," she said. "You decide!"

I switched to the third person. "Let me tell you why some women choose to have this test, and why others don't." Some women did the test for peace of mind, I explained. Some wanted to know of any health problems ahead of time, to be prepared. Others chose to end the pregnancy. Some made arrangements for adoption.

She interrupted me for clarification on adoption. She looked disbelieving when I explained that some parents relinquish their child to another family to raise. "People give their baby away?" she said incredulously. "Why wouldn't they just have an abortion?"

Patients often felt strongly about pregnancy-related choices. I'd had patients who were appalled that someone with a prenatal diagnosis might choose to end the pregnancy;

they accepted their baby's condition as divinely determined, and were opposed to abortion on religious grounds. Others considered it morally reprehensible to knowingly bring a child with a disability into the world. Those with opposing views held them with equal conviction.

I went on to explain why some women chose not to do the blood test: the process caused too much anxiety; they wouldn't risk miscarriage with an amniocentesis in the event of a concerning result; or they would continue the pregnancy under any circumstance.

By watching the patient's reaction as I described the choices others had made, I could usually predict her own decision. This patient was inscrutable, though. I asked what her thoughts were.

The interpreter spoke briefly in Swahili and turned back to me. "So what should she do, Doctor?" I had the impression they were both being patient with me.

I'd done my best to enable her to make an informed decision, although I wondered how much good I'd done. She'd walked into a routine prenatal visit with no concerns, and I'd introduced confusion and reason to worry. She was illiterate, so even if I could find a patient education pamphlet in Swahili, which was unlikely, it wouldn't be useful.

I accepted the responsibility of decision-maker. "Let's do the blood tests," I said.

After printing out the lab requisition I pulled out the Doptone and asked her to lie back on the exam table with her belly exposed. The reassuring sound of baby's heartbeat would put the sobering discussion we'd just had out of her mind. I squeezed some gel onto her abdomen, ran the probe just over her pubic bone, and immediately heard the *whoosh! whoosh! whoosh!* of the fetal heart, 140 beats per minute.

The patient listened in amazement and asked through the interpreter, "That's my baby breathing?"

The afternoon's next patient was Junah. At twenty weeks, she was midway through her pregnancy and this was her last prenatal visit with me. I referred all my obstetrical patients to physicians close to their homes for the second half of pregnancy. With patients scattered across the Lower Mainland, it would be highly impractical for me to attend the deliveries.

We had barely seated ourselves in my little exam room when Junah began to sob. The interpreter listened intently to her concerns, looked aghast, and relayed to me, "The baby has no arms!"

I flipped through the chart for the ultrasound report, certain that I would have recalled signing off on a result with such an unusual anomaly. Sure enough, it read: *Single live fetus. No fetal abnormalities seen today.*

"What makes you think that something is wrong with the baby?" I asked.

Like many of the prenatal patients at the refugee clinic, she had not had an ultrasound in previous pregnancies in her home country and was unfamiliar with the procedure. Apparently, the exam had taken forty minutes, much longer than she had expected, and so she became suspicious that there was a medical concern.

The local radiology departments did not provide interpreters, and most patients did not have an English-speaking friend or family member to accompany them. It wasn't uncommon for a patient to attend the ultrasound appointment alone, unable to ask questions or understand comments, and to follow up with me a week later to review the results with the assistance of the clinic interpreter.

Junah reached into her purse and extracted a printout of an ultrasound image. It was a lateral view of the fetus, with the skull, vertebrae, and protuberant abdomen readily identifiable. She gestured at the picture. "No arms!" she repeated desperately. I could see that to an untrained eye, the baby's upper limbs would indeed appear to be absent.

"The baby does have arms!" I reassured her. "They're not clear in this picture because of how the baby's holding them. Look—I can see the fingers of the right hand over here, and the left shoulder over here." I showed her the corresponding white streaks on the image.

While I enjoyed being an instrument of reassurance, and while it was a pleasure to offer her such enormous relief, it disturbed me that she'd had to navigate the ultrasound experience and its aftermath alone. No mother should have to go a week convinced that her baby has no arms.

The afternoon's final patient was someone I had referred to an obstetrician months before. She was now just six weeks from her due date. The interpreter had called me that morning, concerned, saying that the patient had missed her last appointment with the specialist and refused to return for follow-up. She had indicated that she would be willing to see me, though. Could I talk to her?

I had called the obstetrician's office for information and spoken to the exasperated medical office assistant. "It's urgent," she said. "She needs to be induced for SGA, but she's disappeared." SGA means *small for gestational age*. The baby wasn't growing adequately in utero and needed to be delivered for medical intervention.

"I'll see her this afternoon and see what I can do," I had told the interpreter.

The patient sat across from me now, her belly unusually large for my clinic.

I didn't understand why she would refuse a procedure if her baby's health was in jeopardy, but my policy in the clinic is to never ask a question beginning with *why*. The word implies judgement. It puts patients on the defensive, asking them to explain themselves. "How are you?" I asked. "What's happened?"

"They say they need to take the baby out, because it's so small. But that can't be right. If the baby's too small we should leave it in longer, to let it grow."

No one had taken five minutes to hear her concerns and address them. A fifteen-minute discussion later, I was calling the specialist's office on her behalf to schedule the induction. Clinical acumen and surgical skill counted for next to nothing if you didn't gain the patient's trust and include them in decisions around their care.

25

I PAUSED OUTSIDE THE DOOR TO the exam room, my last minute alone with the terrible news. It felt inequitable, me lingering in the hall with knowledge of her results while she waited patiently in a chair with her purse in her lap, unaware. I did my best to give awful results well, but a soft knock, a turn of the door knob, a few words, and a life would change forever.

The patient was a thirty-four-year-old Congolese woman. She was a community educator from Kisangani, a mother of two, and a widow. She was here to follow up on her screening bloodwork. Her name was Grace.

The results were positive for HIV. I gently told her the diagnosis through the French interpreter. The interpreter looked shaken, struggling to keep her face impartial with tears in her eyes, but the patient said little. I confirmed that she understood what HIV was.

"Yes. She cared for many people who died of it back home," said the interpreter.

HIV treatment and prognosis were different in Canada than in her village, I explained. "With medication and regular doctor visits, most people in Canada with HIV live long, productive lives." It felt like a platitude; it could hardly compete with what she'd seen and heard and smelled in Kisangani.

I'd given many HIV diagnoses over the years, and Grace's stoicism was unusual. I asked how her husband had died. Pneumonia, she told me. He was thirty-two years old. Did he have HIV? I asked. No, pneumonia, she repeated.

"Have you ever been told you have HIV?" I asked. Refugee patients often did not volunteer medical information that was clearly relevant by Canadian standards. I'd learned to ask questions point blank.

"Yes," she said softly. "In the Congo, last year. But I didn't believe them."

I swiftly dispelled that hope. I showed her the lab results: The Western blot and confirmatory tests were positive, and her viral load was 16,000 copies/mL. "The lab triple-checked your results," I told her. "There's no doubt about your diagnosis."

Her CD4 levels, the immune cells attacked by the virus, were just below the normal range at 350 cells/μL. The rest of her labs, including kidney and liver tests, were normal. She felt well and her physical exam was unremarkable, with no sign of opportunistic infection.

"Even though you feel well right now, it's best to start antiretroviral medications," I advised. "It will slow the progression of the infection." I reviewed the options for treatment.

She shook her head. "No. No medication." I waited to hear

her concerns. Did she need information about side effects, or to be reassured that the medications were covered? Then she said the words for which I had no argument: "I believe in miracles," she said with quiet confidence. "Jesus will cure me."

From the age of six, I pushed my sister to school in an oversized stroller. Julia is thirteen months older than me. While she could use a walker, the three blocks to school were too much for a seven-year-old with cerebral palsy.

We shared an upstairs bedroom in our small home in Burnaby. After our dad had read the story of Peter healing the lame man from the children's Bible after dinner one night, Julia and I prayed in our beds for our own miracle. We decided to give God the night to do His work. In the morning I watched as she stiffly moved her feet from the bed onto the rug. She pushed herself to standing, wobbled, and attempted her first step. She toppled to the floor, right arm contracted tightly against her body.

Our prayers hadn't worked, and I knew the reason from the nightly Bible stories: my faith wasn't strong enough. I suspected my impure motivation was a factor, too. I desperately wanted Julia to walk, but I also wanted the importance of bursting into the kitchen and telling my parents the best news of their lives. Jesus could heal her, I was certain. He simply wouldn't, and that was my fault, not His.

That was my view on miracles well into adulthood: they could happen, but they didn't, and they wouldn't. I must have been thirty-five when I finally acknowledged that perhaps this meant I didn't believe in miracles at all. But plenty of people around me did.

"The eighteen-week ultrasound showed cysts in her brain," one of my friends said at a birthday party that weekend, bouncing her six-month-old on her hip. "But everyone prayed for her during the rest of the pregnancy and she was born perfectly healthy. A miracle." There were appreciative murmurs from the guests.

Spontaneous resolution of a choroid plexus cyst, I corrected her, silently. They occurred in 1 to 2 percent of pregnancies, and almost always disappeared on their own. I took another sip of wine and kept quiet. Everybody loves a miracle. I wasn't about to be the spoilsport.

Over the years, I'd quietly dismissed every account of a healing miracle I'd encountered. Every story told to me had to have a medical explanation. What others attributed to miracles I assigned to chemotherapy, rehabilitation, natural course of illness. Others invoked the supernatural when they could not explain something, or were desperate.

Medicine continually seeks explanation; writing something off as a miracle flies in the face of the purpose of scientific research. There's plenty in medicine that is not currently understood, but will be eventually, with the advancement of science.

And so I didn't encourage Grace with the story of another of my HIV-positive patients, an Eritrean woman who also refused treatment, and whose viral load remained undetectable for years, regardless. That patient so puzzled me that I retested her for HIV, and called the microbiologist wondering if it might be a false positive. It wasn't, he assured me. Some might call her a miracle, but we called her a non-progressor. We didn't know why she wasn't deteriorating, but we were certain there was a reason. It just hadn't been discovered yet.

When Grace told me she was forgoing emtricitabine,

tenofovir, and efavirenz in favour of divine healing, I didn't protest, at least not outwardly. She wasn't asking me for a miracle, or even expecting me to believe in one. She'd simply confided her own intentions to me. I didn't want to spook her with arguments; I wanted her to continue to come to see me.

"Let's check your blood again in two months," I suggested. "Come back then and we'll review your CD4 and viral load."

"They will be better next time," she said. She spoke with conviction. Her smile was serene. I could see something beautiful in her belief, but I couldn't have shared it even if I'd wanted to. And I'm not sure she wanted me to. It would be unnerving, I think, to learn that one's doctor relied on supernatural intervention to treat patients.

"I hope so," I told her. My pragmatic thoughts slunk to the fore. I only hoped the inevitable downward drift would be slow enough that I'd have enough time to convince her to put her hope in reverse transcriptase inhibitors.

In six weeks, her viral load had not dropped but her CD4 count increased to 380 cells/μL. Given that a fluctuation of 30 percent in a day is still within the normal range, I didn't put much stock in the value. But Grace did.

"I wondered whether to ask the church to pray for me," she confided, her quiet voice as excited as I'd heard it. "But I didn't want the whole community to know. Jesus heard my prayers, though." She was buoyant.

Two months later, the level dipped to 340 cells/μL. This was not a significant change from baseline, but Grace was deflated. She resolved to pray more. I told her that Atripla could be taken once daily with minimal side effects. She smiled at my persistence, me of little faith, and reminded me: "I trust in Jesus."

For months Grace's CD4 bobbed gently around 350 cells/μL, and we bobbed in place, too. At every visit, she reported her religious practices, and I reported her lab results. Each small dip was followed by a spike, so that her hopes were renewed. We weren't going anywhere.

Then I learned that she had a new partner.

"Did you tell him that you're HIV positive?" I asked. She hadn't. She didn't want word to leak out to the African community in Vancouver.

"Are you using condoms?"

"Sometimes."

It was one thing to accommodate her hope for a miracle, but it was another to put others at risk while we waited. HIV non-disclosure is a criminal act in Canada. "You need to tell him," I urged. "And you must use a condom every time you have sex."

She nodded and said nothing for a minute. Then, in her soft voice, "He won't use condoms, even when I tell him to." After a pause, "I'm afraid to tell him about my HIV. I'm afraid he will hurt me."

We talked about safety, and her options. We talked about healthy relationships. And then I doggedly brought up treatment, again. "Perhaps Jesus could work through the medication," I tried.

She thought about that. "Maybe."

Six weeks later she changed her mind without fanfare. "I ended my relationship," she told me. I'd barely tasted the relief when she continued, simply, "I'm ready to start the medication."

We looked at each other. How strange that this moment of her loosening her dependence on the divine could feel so holy. I said only, "Yes." I sent in the Atripla prescription and arranged an appointment with the pharmacist.

When I saw her next, her viral load had plummeted from 16,000 to 250 copies/mL.

"Praise God," she said when I gave her the good news. "Thank you, Jesus."

And then, after an appropriate pause, "Thank you, Dr. Scholtens."

26

"Do you think you'll return to journalism?" I asked Yusef. "Once your English has improved?"

Through the Resettlement Assistance Program, the Haddads received federal funding for their first year in Canada, while they settled into their community and learned English. The family lived on $1,350 a month. Now that the first year was almost over, Yusef was expected to find employment.

"My English will never be good enough. I will never have the fluency." He stated this matter-of-factly, almost hiding his sorrow. "First, a job. Then maybe find a better job or work my way up. Every job wants Canadian work experience, though."

He was delivering his resume to electronics warehouses on King George Highway and pizzerias in Whalley. Even educated refugees typically started at jobs requiring physical labour and minimal English, such as warehouse work, construction at the new SkyTrain terminals in Coquitlam, or painting houses. I hadn't often considered the human hands doing the menial work behind the scenes of everyday life, but after my fifty-year-old Myanmar patient found work packing cucumbers into boxes eight hours a day, I thought of her every time I saw neatly packed cartons of produce at the grocery store.

Six weeks before, Yusef had shown up at the walk-in clinic to request the medication I'd previously mentioned as a potential treatment for post-traumatic stress disorder. I'd given him a prescription for sertraline, with instructions on how to titrate it over the first few weeks. Since then he had waved off any discussion of his symptoms, except to assure me that he was "much better." He wanted to talk about his job search.

"Did you bring your medication?" I asked. I encouraged patients to bring all their prescriptions to every visit. The proportion of patients who took them as prescribed approached zero. It was much easier to review medications with the pills in hand than to discuss *the small round white pill.*

He pulled a sheet of blister-packed pills from his bag. The days of the week were printed down the left side, and four plastic bubbles ran next to each day, from left to right: BREAKFAST, LUNCH, DINNER, BEDTIME. Patients accessed the pills by punching out the foil at the back of the compartment. Dispensing medications this way improved compliance for most patients, but for newcomers to Canada the system wasn't necessarily intuitive, especially for patients who read from right to left, as Yusef did in Arabic. I looked over the sheet he handed me. The compartments for the previous few days were empty. A yellow and white capsule and small white tablet rattled in each of the breakfast bubbles for the remaining days of the week. I nodded and passed it back to him.

If Yusef wouldn't talk about his mental health directly, I took this new focus on employment as a surrogate marker. It was reassuring. Freud suggested that two hallmarks of a healthy life are the abilities to love and to work: *lieben und arbeiten*.[1] I considered work not just a marker of health but a means to achieve it. Aside from the obvious benefits of income and extended health insurance, employment provided dignity, structure, and a social network. It offered an opportunity to learn English and distraction from personal difficulties. Work was therapy.

One of my patients was a twenty-three-year-old Eastern European refugee claimant who worked at McDonalds. She took her job very seriously as she depended on it to pay the legal fees to the lawyer representing her asylum claim. She had to contend with past trauma, the stress of preparing her case, and an unknown future. She folded in on herself under the pressure and kept to herself at work.

At the start of her shift one morning her manager told her, "I need to talk to you at the end of the day." Her heart sank. The day dragged on, and when she finally met with her boss that afternoon, her fears were confirmed when he began, "Your co-workers have approached me with some concerns. They've noticed that you seem worried and withdrawn, that you don't join in when they're joking around and having fun. They want to know if there's anything they can do to help you feel more relaxed." No prescription could compete with a thoughtful manager and supportive group of coworkers at a fast-food restaurant.

"I brought mail," Yusef said now. He unclipped his satchel and pulled out a bundle of envelopes. This was not unusual. Patients often brought me mail that confused them, especially government and legal letters. I had mixed feelings about this. Reading someone else's mail felt voyeuristic, an intense breach of privacy. But it often included information on medical appointments or health insurance, and I was grateful for a chance to intercept these.

"This one is from TB Control," I said, refolding the pink tissue sheet and reinserting it into the envelope. "Your chest X-ray was clear and you don't need to go back." Yusef made a note on the envelope in Arabic.

"This one confirms that you're enrolled with British Columbia's Medical Services Plan. Keep it for your records."

The third letter was a fare infraction notice from TransLink. "This is a fine for riding SkyTrain without a ticket," I said.

"I thought I would pay the conductor on the train." SkyTrain stations did not have ticket turnstiles. I could understand how he might have moved with throngs of commuters with monthly passes down the stairs of King George Station onto the platform, unaware that he had to purchase a ticket from the machines off to the side at the station entrance.

"There is no conductor. You have to purchase a ticket before getting on the train," I said. "This fine is for $173.00." Yusef asked me to repeat this, twice. It was an inconceivable amount to him. I read the fine print. The ticket could be disputed within fourteen days. The notice was stamped a month previous.

"I'll write a letter on your behalf," I said, turning to my computer. "You can bring or mail it to the address on the letter." Typing rapidly, I explained his error, his situation, his income.

I asked for mercy, for a reduction or waiving of the fine. Yusef waited patiently, appreciatively. I didn't go to medical school to read mail for people and petition TransLink to forgive fines, but it was these practical interventions that seemed to mean the most to patients.

I'd been asked before by confused patients if I was a social worker. *No, but I'm going to address your homelessness, finances, or food security first, everything else second.* Pulling an extra $200 from this month's meagre budget would impact Yusef's health, whether by increasing tension in the household, reducing the grocery budget, or restricting his ability to pay the bus fare to come to the clinic or attend job interviews.

I signed the letter, handed it to Yusef, and wished him luck. He was grateful, but I couldn't help wondering if a simpler solution would have been to quietly pay the fine myself.

Sometimes I fantasized about anonymously mailing patients an envelope stuffed with cash. I imagined the relief that such a windfall could give, although a random wad of hundred dollar bills arriving in the mail could be construed as ominous. I couldn't do a mail-out to my entire patient roster, so I'd have to be selective about the recipients, and that was ethically fraught. Financial dealings with patients violated the codes of the College of Physicians and Surgeons of BC, of course. I pictured the write-up in the back of its quarterly newsletter, in the Disciplinary Actions section. Then again, a doctor slipping money to her patients might be a welcome break from the usual stories of fraudulent billings and sexual misconduct.

I resisted the temptation to give patients money. The closest I came was when I diagnosed a Sudanese musician with depression. I knew that what he needed more than any prescription or counselling was a piano. I saw a beautiful one at the thrift store and considered having it delivered to him, benefactor unknown. He lived in a fourth-floor walk-up, though, and I gave up the idea when I considered the delivery logistics. I made the right decision, per my professional regulatory body. I'm not sure my patient would agree. That piano might have saved a life.

In his book *Walden,* Henry David Thoreau notes that our money goes first to meeting the basic needs of warmth, shelter, food, and clothing.[2] He marvels that once those needs are met, rather than turning our attention to more interesting and important issues, we devote ourselves to attaining bigger shelter, finer food, and a more fashionable wardrobe. I thought of this often, as I witnessed extremes of wealth and poverty in my professional life.

I worked in one of the least lucrative corners of medicine. I didn't own a condo in Whistler or take the kids to Europe in the summer; we drove a Honda minivan and our kitchen fixtures were from the seventies. But I had more than enough—enough to purchase an Eames chair, an iconic bent plywood piece with a broad curved seat set low to the ground. It was delivered that fall with a Herman Miller certificate of authenticity. It was the first piece of fine furniture I owned.

The next day at the clinic, as I gave a young mother instruction on how to access the Food Bank, the beautiful chair came to mind. It was worth the equivalent of three or four months of groceries for her family. As I left the clinic on my lunch break to get a sandwich from Terra Breads, I noticed a colleague's Audi A7 in the clinic parking lot. It made the purchase of the chair seem reasonable, briefly. It made the disparity of wealth in society seem enormous.

At the bistro, I paid \$8.60 for a grilled asiago cheese sandwich on sourdough bread and \$3.00 for an Americano. My lunch would be a financial indulgence for every patient I'd seen that morning. In fact, most of my life was lived in relative luxury: I never ran into patients at my usual out-of-office haunts—the Mt Seymour ski hill, the *Nutcracker* at the Queen Elizabeth Theatre, the upscale Pidgin Restaurant.

When I did, it was jarring. Deep Cove is a tourist attraction. Mountains hulk over the seaside village, centred on a one-street strip lined with bistros and art galleries that dead-ends onto a stunning viewpoint of the cove. When I see visitors admiring the view, I feel as proud as if I'd created it myself.

Every second night, I run. I run through the woods, mindful of tree roots, cougar warnings, and owls that swoop in the dusk. I run along the waterfront, past the kayak rental, the dock, and the red lifeguard chair on its long thin legs. While running that stretch I can never resist swivelling my head to the right, admiring the little harbour golden in the evening light, and the glittering green jetty wrapping around it. I loop back home through quiet back lanes.

Running makes me feel like an animal in the most wonderful way. My work is relational and cerebral, but running reduces me to a biological creature, moving, breathing, sweating. I flop onto the grass at the beach and feel my ribcage thudding against the damp earth. I am a living creature that will die. But not just yet.

One evening as I pounded past the kayak rental centre, I came across Yusef kneeling on a prayer mat on the beach. His eyes were closed. I had no idea what etiquette dictated in this situation. Should I wait and greet him? I decided to continue.

A hundred metres later I saw Junah, Nadia, and Layth approaching from the dock. They saw me before I could sprint away.

I was wearing a purple sports bra with a light blue running tank, spandex tights, and pink Nikes. My hair was pulled back in a sweat-soaked headband. When I saw that they recognized me, I stopped and pulled out my earbuds. I hoped my attire wasn't offensive to them.

They looked extremely interested in what I was doing, and formed an attentive half circle around me. "You live here, Doctor?"

"Yes!" I gestured at the treed point forming the south curve of the cove, studded with houses hanging onto cliffs.

"So beautiful!"

"Yes. It is." Sweat trickled down my bare, freckled shoulders. I felt exposed.

"Have a good night, Doctor."

I jogged off, heading for home with the sun slanting through the cedars and raindrops in white relief in the flare. At least I was modelling healthy activity, I thought. Although when I'd discussed exercise with the Haddads in the past, I'd learned that they couldn't afford athletic shoes.

27

IOWA CITY HAD FRAT HOUSES, American flags hanging over front porches, and bunnies running across lawns. The place was unpretentious and friendly. I was in town for a narrative medicine conference, three days of immersion in words and ideas at the Carver College of Medicine.

"Take a year to read forty novels and one hundred short stories," the first speaker advised us. "You'll have the equivalent of an MFA." The idea seemed to hold universal appeal for the audience. We represented everything from pediatric cardiology to social work to public health, but we all loved to read and write.

"Physicians ought to write," said another lecturer, physician-writer Dr. Louise Aronson, "for three reasons: to reflect, to memorialize, and to advocate." This mirrored physicians' triple obligation to self, patient, and society, she suggested.

I felt convicted. I had done the first two tasks unprompted, for years, but I had little interest in the third.

The advocates I'd encountered struck me as bitter and shrill. Social justice felt like a fad, something to which people flocked to feel morally superior. I was an introvert with no political savvy. I didn't want to publicly champion a cause. I just wanted to see patients in my exam room, with the door closed, during office hours.

I admired religious and medical pragmatism, though, and advocacy for my patients fit with both. My patients were vulnerable. They were rendered effectively voiceless, either by a language barrier or by terrible personal experiences with protests. When federal health insurance for refugees was slashed months after the Iowa conference, I was in a unique position to see what the cuts looked like on the ground. They looked awful: unfair, unsafe, impractical, and short-sighted. Clearly someone had to speak up. I realized, with some reluctance, that that someone was me.

I wrote an editorial, urging British Columbia to fill in the gaps for refugee health coverage. This time, I followed the advice that Dr. Aronson had given at the conference: *Humanize someone who is unlike the reader. Make it personal. No jargon. No more than three pieces of data. Know what you want.*

> Leila is a thirty-four-year-old Iranian woman with asthma severe enough that it has landed her in the intensive care unit on two occasions. Her asthma is well managed now, after years of having her medications tweaked by her doctors in Tehran. She rummages in her purse and lines up three inhalers

on my desk, each with a different coloured cap, labelled in Farsi script. She needs a refill.

There's one problem. She's a refugee claimant in British Columbia.

The Interim Federal Health Program, funded by Citizenship and Immigration Canada, has provided limited, temporary health insurance to refugees since 1957. The program has recently been slashed. Refugees are now stratified by category, status, and country of origin, and health-insurance packages doled out accordingly. The lucky ones get close to the original coverage for their first few months in the country. The unluckiest get care only if they put Canadians at risk.

Leila arrived in Vancouver last month and has a hearing date in a few weeks. She has IFH coverage, but it excludes all medications. IFH will pay for any number of emergency room visits, an ICU admission, and a consult by a respirologist but it will not cover a Ventolin puffer.

There's a small supply of medication in our clinic cupboard reserved for emergencies. I give her two puffers, which don't match the lineup on my desk, and a prescription for the original medications. It's the best I can do. She'll have to find the money to fill her prescription, somehow, even though she's told me that when the family travels three SkyTrain fare zones to the clinic, they eat less for dinner. Maybe a church group will help her, or there'll be a pharmaceutical sample in the cupboard next time. I explain how to call 911.

Why has the government of BC been completely silent on the issue of health insurance for refugees in this province? It's time to clean up this mess, even if we didn't make it. I'm asking our leaders in BC to join the other provinces in committing to ensuring that all refugees have access to care.[1]

I recommended some specific measures that the government could take that would improve the situation. The *Province* newspaper promptly published the op-ed. Next to the article was a picture of me that I thought alarmingly prominent. I felt exposed. I appreciated the support on social media, especially by my academic family at UBC and colleagues working in refugee medicine, but I dreaded the inevitable pushback.

The next day I read the letters to the editor in response to my article, most of which protested the restoration of healthcare insurance for refugees. Then I shared the responses with my kids. They had proudly brought the article to school, and I thought that they ought to see the other side of speaking up.

"Here's what Andy Baker of Chilliwack had to say," I told them. They waited expectantly. "'Dr. Martina Scholtens' op-ed is, to put it mildly, disgusting.'"

Saskia's jaw dropped. "But Mom! Did anyone like it?" This wasn't about being liked, I told them. It was about making people pay attention. And the next day Terry Lake, the Minister of Health, wrote in to the *Province* to respond. He defended the existing system: "The B.C. government takes its humanitarian responsibilities seriously. The first priority for the health system is always that patients receive the care they need. We will not deny or turn away anyone from essential services in an acute care setting."

I hadn't expected change overnight. Action would take months or years. Bringing awareness to the issue was just the first step.

A few weeks later, I helped organize the Day of Action healthcare worker protest to be held in Vancouver, a few blocks from Pete's Yaletown office. "I'll walk over during my lunch break," Pete told me the night before. "Will there be speakers?"

"Yes. Me, for one," I answered.

"You're kidding."

I wasn't. I'd even bought a new white coat with a Peter Pan collar for the occasion.

The crowd gathered in front of the Immigration and Refugee Board office. There were colleagues from the refugee clinic, physicians from St. Paul's Hospital, nurses, midwives, passersby, and, at the edge of the group, a handful of curious patients.

When one of my patients had mentioned that he might attend, I worried that his PTSD might be triggered by seeing law enforcement. I warned him that police would likely be present.

"Why?" He was alarmed.

"Just to keep everyone safe. To make sure no one falls off the sidewalk onto the street."

In months of weekly encounters, I'd never seen him smile, but at this description of police work he had laughed in amazement.

"My name is Martina Scholtens, and I'm a family doctor," I told the crowd. "One of the basic tenets of medicine is, 'First, do no harm.' Whether you do clinical care, work on a population level, or develop government healthcare, that ought to be a guiding principle." I invited the crowd to repeat the phrase throughout my speech.

I told the crowd of an eight-year-old Iranian boy whose life-saving medication wasn't covered by the new federal health insurance structure.

"Do no harm!" chanted the crowd.

I told the story of a Mexican child who had neither his medications, specialist visits, nor hospital admissions covered.

"Do no harm!"

I talked about the financial costs of the cuts to hospitals and taxpayers. I pointed out that newly arrived refugees were future Canadian citizens—our future colleagues, children's classmates, and neighbours, and that we ought to be investing in them. Only treating disease that threatened the Canadian public was degrading; putting patients in the position where they had to beg for medications was humiliating.

"Do no harm!"

Healthcare should not be used as political leverage in immigration policy, and the dignity of my patients was not dispensable.

"Do no harm!"

Then I raced back to the clinic in time for my first afternoon patient. It was Yusef.

"I heard you on the radio this morning," he said. I'd been on CBC's *Early Edition* with Rick Cluff. Yusef marvelled that I could publicly disagree with the government without fear of repercussions. "We want to say thank you, for your help," he went on.

I was surprised by how closely he had followed our campaign. While I had seen advocacy as distinct from direct clinical care of the patient, something I did off the side of my desk, it was clear that Yusef saw it differently.

"We have made you a Facebook fan page in Arabic," he said.

28

I FIRST FELT THE BABY MOVE at sixteen weeks: a soft swipe, a sliding sensation. Then the movements changed to knocks, small thuds, bumps, and turns. I often lay on the couch, pants unbuttoned, both hands on my belly, waiting for baby to buck and shift; its solid presence took my breath away.

At twenty-seven weeks, three days, I had a globe of a belly, a baby cardigan on the knitting needles, three very pleased children, and a nonstop pace at the office that kept baby rocked to sleep most of the day.

I disliked that pregnancy forced me to bring my personal life into the office. I didn't have pictures of my kids on my desk, I was vague when curious patients asked where I lived, and on Monday mornings I never volunteered my weekend activities to the staff. But my pregnant belly, no matter how discreetly swathed in muted professional clothes, begged comment from everybody.

When a patient came to see me for a follow-up after a miscarriage, I was acutely aware how difficult it might be for her to see her doctor pregnant. As I called her from the waiting room I felt I was flaunting my fertility. I willed my belly to shrink down a little, to look less jaunty, but her gaze was fixed on it as she approached. She grabbed my arm, looked at me earnestly, and said, "I'm happy for you. I really am." I could tell she was, and I was moved by her graciousness.

Not everyone was happy for me. I had lunch with a colleague in town for a conference, a forty-something man with no children, and he asked what benefits I received as a member of our provincial medical association. I listed them: malpractice insurance rebates, education funding, maternity leave benefits . . .

He interrupted me. "Why should others pay for your lifestyle choice?" He gave a short diatribe on the injustices borne by childless men. I tried to interject but gave up when he complained about having to pay taxes for neighbourhood schools, which didn't benefit him directly.

"If you get a leave to have a baby, I should get paid leave to take a watercolour painting course," he concluded.

A few days later he swung by my office on his way to the airport. He set a steaming coffee on my desk and offered contritely, "You can have as many children as you want, Martina." It wasn't an apology for his position, I knew; it was an effort to mend the damage done to our friendship by articulating it.

I began my maternity leave a week before my due date. I waited impatiently at home, hovering between two worlds—missing the clinic, and not yet consumed by the newborn days. The baby was born two long days past the due date.

I included the requisite statistics on the birth announcement. I was precise, to the gram, the minute. What I cared about, though, in the days after her birth, were the other details. That my semi-retired doctor came up from a day at his cabin digging a garden for raspberry canes, for his last delivery. The warm blankets piled on me postpartum, white flannel with pink and blue stripes, the softness gone after hundreds of launderings—how they reminded me so strongly of both nights on call in the same hospital and my previous deliveries. The red birthmarks on my newborn daughter's eyelids, symmetrical flames, perfect.

"Raspberry canes? Those are just the hormones talking," said my girlfriend flatly. Maybe it was. Did it matter what magnified the incidental facts around her birth? I was still sifting through the experience, letting the details settle. I didn't have any perspective yet, and I was hardly coherent.

Before I left the hospital, the public health liaison took a history from me and asked after my occupation. "I'm a family doctor at a refugee clinic," I said, and I was almost startled to hear myself say it, as if I'd suddenly remembered it. I turned away as tears came. Hormones and lack of sleep, yes—and a sudden brief nostalgia for a life that seemed to have very rapidly receded. Most of all, though, the grateful realization, as I sat cross-legged in the hospital bed with my infant daughter in my lap, considering my work, was that *I have this—and I have* that, *too*.

I felt rich. Three daughters and a son. And I felt unified with my patients. I thought about how the process of birth is fundamentally the same the world over: pain, mess, relief and, if we are lucky, joy. I thought of Junah, just months from delivery, and imagined her with her prize in her arms, the baby wearing the same white flannel gown and yellow knit hat as my daughter.

We named our daughter Ilia Tove. Several times in the first week the entire family spontaneously migrated to her room, forming an admiring semicircle around her crib. Her siblings adored her. "Hey Ilia!" said Leif the first time he met her, waving his hands gently in her face. "Dynamite!" and his fingers burst apart in a soft explosion. Ariana imitated her startle reflex perfectly. And Saskia pored over my baby books: "Mom! Did you know that in a few months you can mash up a banana and feed it to her?" Pete walked around with a pink flannel burp cloth over his right shoulder, ready to soothe the baby that looked just like him.

Ilia attended three show-and-tells during her first week. "She breastfeeds," Leif told his Grade 1 class. "She breastfeeds breast milk. From my mom's breasts." He patted my right breast for good measure. "All her life, my mom's body has been saving all the milk she ever drank to feed this baby," he went on knowledgeably. "It even saved all the milk my mom drank as a little girl."

When Ilia was a few weeks old, Pete asked casually from the couch where he was reading after dinner, "Do you miss our old life?" The relief to hear it said! I did. I missed the old routine, driving in to Vancouver in the mornings with four-year-old Ariana in the back seat, CBC on the radio, and a day at the clinic ahead of me. Yes, there would be a similar routine in a few months, with an infant in the car and a gradual return to work, but those other days, with their own particular details about which I was already sentimental, were done.

"I guess you'll never have another son-baby, hey, Mom?"

Leif asked cheerfully as he ate his after-school snack the next week. I could have cried. I had saved all my kids' clothes in anticipation of this possible fourth, and now that she'd arrived I had boxes of corduroy pants, sneakers, and little ball caps to set afloat. Somehow my daughters' infancies seemed preserved through newborn Ilia wearing their hand-me-downs, but I couldn't kid myself: my son's baby days were over.

And then I overheard Ariana greeting her little sister. "Good morning, Ilia," she said seriously. "It's your medium-sized sister." Saskia was still the oldest, and Leif was still the only boy, but the crown of youngest child had been passed from Ariana to Ilia, by my choice. Then, after church, an elderly woman tugged on my arm, admired the baby and confided, "Mothers have a very special relationship with their youngest daughter." At that moment Ariana came into view with her long dark pigtails, her thin legs in purple boots making their way across the room to the gardens outside. There she was, the daughter with whom I would have had that extra special relationship—except I'd taken that from us and given it to this newest baby.

Those first two months, I missed my bodies. The one before this last pregnancy. The one before I had ever been pregnant at all. The pregnant one, even; that at least looked purposeful. A week postpartum, sitting at the breakfast table, Leif gestured at my paunch with his spoon and asked, "You know why that looks like that? Because all the equipment is still in there."

Most of all, I struggled with the loss of my identity as physician. At the little goodbye party over cake in the chart room in November, I had asked the clinic to please just stagnate until I returned. Of course, I expected them to forge ahead and do all sorts of interesting things while I was away, and I hated to not be a part of it. Some of my patients, like Yusef, requested four-month supplies of medications to tide them over until my return. I didn't comply, but I understood. I was grateful for the locum covering for me in my absence, but I was jealous of her, too. I missed the collegiality of the clinic, the focus on others' lives, the escape from my own head, the sense of contributing to the community, the academic stimulation. I'd be back to work in the spring, but in the meantime, I felt unmoored.

Yet how I loved my daughter's little face. I marvelled that someone I couldn't have imagined months ago could feel so inevitable, could have an entire family happily orbiting around her. My sorrow was not ingratitude. It was simply an acknowledgment that for this new mother, mixed in with the bliss of those first six to eight weeks, were feelings of loss and grief.

29

I RETURNED TO WORK WHEN ILIA was four months old. Yusef was booked to see me on my first day back. We traded details on our babies. Ahmed was a month old. Yusef showed me pictures on his phone of Junah cradling a baby with fuzzed black hair and wide eyes so dark they swallowed his pupils. "He's beautiful," I said, but I was looking at Junah. She smiled with her lips closed, serene, all weariness gone from her face, lifting her elbow to tip Ahmed toward the camera.

Upon returning from maternity leave, I'd promptly looked up Junah's file to read the delivery report and newborn assessment. It had been a spontaneous vaginal delivery at thirty-nine weeks, I read, scanning the report, and the baby's exam was normal. She'd taken risks that I had not advised, and the result was an uneventful pregnancy and an eight-pound seven-ounce healthy son.

The family doctor in Surrey who had provided care for Junah's last four months of pregnancy and attended the delivery had agreed to take on the Haddads as patients. We were a few months past their one-year anniversary in Canada, when I usually discharged patients from the clinic. Today was Yusef's last visit with me.

"Party for Junah's birthday," Yusef said carefully at the end of the visit, with his Arabic accent. "You come, Doctor?"

He sat in the patient chair to the left of my desk, long legs crossed, shoes shined. There was no interpreter. Eager to practice his English, and, I suspected, to optimize the intimacy of the visit, he now declined Hani's assistance and insisted on seeing me alone.

It was mid-afternoon, and I was cheerful and unguarded on my first day back. "I don't know," I said as I printed his prescription. "When is it?"

He seized on this suggestion of interest. "You come? Junah so happy! I tell her Doctor come."

"Well, I don't know if I can make it," I said. "What day is it?"

"You tell the day you can come," he said.

That felt all wrong, organizing a birthday party around the doctor's availability. I refused to name a date.

"I choose date," Yusef said agreeably. "I email you. You cannot come, I change date." He gathered his coat and umbrella and murmured again as he left the exam room, "Junah so happy when I tell her."

I'd never been invited to a patient's birthday party, but I already felt uneasy. Had this been an exam question during my medical training, I would have stated with certainty that attendance would be unprofessional.

But when I thought about the actual practice of physicians I admired, it was less clear. A Vancouver obstetrician hosted an annual party at her home for the new parents, with a legendary Bellini machine. My father-in-law golfed with his physician. My own family doctor listed his home address publicly, to ensure he'd always be available to patients. All of the above seemed unprofessional in theory, but reasonable in practice. Noble, even.

The next day Yusef emailed me at my work address. The line spacing was odd, and he had clearly used a translation service; the effect was poetic:

Hello my doctor,

First, thank you for everything.

We came to the most beautiful city in the world
before more than a year.
From the first day you was balm for us
and eased the pain of alienation.
We always see you as more than a doctor for us
we consider you a close friend.

Doctor, for all of this and other
we will be very happy if you accepted
the invitation to celebrate Junah's birthday
on Sunday March 10 at 4 PM.

From there he detailed an elaborate itinerary that involved touring the city of Surrey in his friend's car and visiting White

Rock beach before returning to his home for the birthday party.

I was moved by his invitation—and I resented it. I didn't want to be a special guest. I was the host, in my exam room.

I strove for a professional but cordial reply. A relationship with a physician, I told him, was special, with limitations on how we could engage outside the clinic. I declined the city tour and beach visit, but would try to come by the house briefly during the party to give my regards to Junah. I hoped he understood, I concluded.

He replied immediately: "Yes, yes, of course, Doctor."

The Surrey address was a few minutes off the freeway, on a street where everyone drove by hurriedly on their way somewhere else. It was a neighbourhood of low apartment buildings, with old couches and bikes on the balconies and scrappy lawns. As I approached, I slowed uncertainly, trying to make out the address numbers in the winter dark. Then I saw Yusef at the parking entrance, waving at me. I pulled in and rolled down my window.

Yusef welcomed me with formality, and directed me where to park. He wore a suit jacket and cologne. I was deliberately dressed exactly as I did for the clinic: navy wool pants, a blouse in a small print, and low heels. Only the stethoscope draped around my neck was missing. Business attire was unimaginative, but festive dress felt downright dangerous. I was determined to preserve some kind of boundary.

We walked into the building together. I knew that most of my patient demographic lived in poverty, but I had never actually witnessed it. The halls were dim, and garbage was piled next to the doors of some units. I could taste something sour—stale cigarette smoke, or cat urine. Had I been alone I would have felt unsafe.

Upstairs, Yusef ushered me into his apartment. I entered the living room, dull beige, unadorned except for a row of plants crowded in the windowsill, and harshly lit by an unshaded bulb hanging from the ceiling. In the centre of the room was a table loaded with food. Next to it stood Junah, smiling shyly, with makeup on and the bundled baby in her arms. Nadia and Layth were lined up beside her.

A man and a woman stood up from the loveseat and introduced themselves. They appeared Middle Eastern but their English was fluent. They had met Junah and Yusef two weeks earlier at the local high school, they told me. We were the only guests.

I wished Junah a happy birthday, and good health in the coming year. I presented her with a small kalanchoe plant wrapped in green foil that I'd picked up from Safeway on the way over. I'd had to choose between two discomforts: buying a gift for a patient or showing up at a party empty-handed. The plant was well-received.

So was I. I sat on the couch, and Junah and Yusef sat on chairs opposite me and beamed at me. I was clearly the guest of honour.

Yusef spoke in Arabic to the other guests, who turned and looked at me. "So you're their doctor?" asked the man doubtfully.

"Yes."

"I've never heard of a doctor going to a patient's birthday party," he said.

"They typically don't," I said. He waited, but I had nothing more to say.

We sat in silence. Never at a loss for words in the clinic, I could think of nothing to say. I already knew the intimate details of their lives, down to their monthly budget and what they dreamed about at night. In the office, nothing was off-limits. Here, nothing seemed appropriate.

"I show you house?" asked Yusef.

"Yes, please." I followed him through the apartment. The kitchen was warm and savoury, the dishes from food preparation piled on the counter. The master bedroom contained nothing but a double bed. Nadia and Layth shared the second bedroom. There were no sheets on the mattresses, just a rumpled blanket on each one. The single bathroom was so small that it would be awkward for a lone occupant to close the door.

I thought back over various conversations I'd had with the Haddads in the clinic, and retrofitted them into the context of this apartment. I matched the insomnia to the bed, the trouble concentrating on homework to the shared bedroom, and the loneliness to the anonymous Surrey apartment complex. The family had been in clear focus for me in the clinic, the rest of their life a blurred abstract. They lived here, though—not in my exam room.

"Eat!" Yusef commanded when we returned to the living room. It took me three servings to realize that clearing the plate indicated that I was still hungry, and signalled Junah to heap it with more dumplings and date-and-sesame balls. I finally tried setting it down with a few forkfuls of food remaining, and my hosts nodded with satisfaction.

Shortly after, the other two guests excused themselves. I wanted to follow suit, but it hadn't even been an hour since I'd arrived. With my departure, the celebration would be over. I remained seated on the couch and sipped the tea Junah served.

After a few minutes of silence Yusef left the room and returned with a flat cardboard box the size of his hand. He set it on the coffee table, shook off the lid, and pushed the box toward me. Inside was a stack of photos. They were smaller than the standard four-by-six-inch Canadian prints, with rounded corners.

I laughed with delight at the top one, an image of a much younger Yusef, with the lean build and unapologetic hair of a man in his twenties, leaning over the open hood of a car. The next was of an extraordinarily pudgy baby whose distinct facial characteristics I immediately knew to be Layth's. Beneath this was a photo was of three children, two boys and a girl, seated on a blanket in a shaded courtyard filled with potted plants. These were the pictures the Haddads had brought with them when they fled Iraq, I realized. I went through the entire stack, exclaiming with recognition as I flipped through the catalogue of their life before we met.

The Haddads gathered around me, pleased with my reaction and offering commentary on the different scenes. Yusef sat on one side of me, Junah on the other, and Nadia and Layth leaned on the arms of the couch. Ahmed slept in Junah's lap, his right arm flung up over his head, hand balled into a little fist. His heart was the size of that fist, I thought, tiny but robust, and one day, God willing, it would be the size of his father's. If he were anything like his parents that fist would be one of gripping strength, an antidote to the fists of aggression that had obliterated the life in the box of photos.

An hour later I drove home to the North Shore, eyes drawn to where the silver of the March sky met the dark ridge of the mountains. The magic always seemed to be where two things brushed against each other, I thought. It was why I liked the beach, and conversation, and dusk. In the exam room, too, the patient and I were two eternal spheres that rubbed up against each other, making a little spark to see by. Most was left unknown. It was that thin line where we met that was beautiful.

I pulled up to my weathered 1970s home overlooking the waters of Indian Arm, neighbours obscured by massive cedars, with a minivan in the driveway and bikes strewn across the yard. My home had never seemed so splendid, or so preposterous.

A few days later I received an email from Yusef with a photo attached. The plant I had given Junah was in bloom. The text, poetic as always, had been garbled in translation. I gathered that the flowers reminded them of my visit, and both made them extraordinarily happy.

Every few months I receive a message—usually from a patient, often stripped of the subtleties afforded by fluency in English—that reminds me why I am a family doctor. I read Yusef's email twice, tagged it DON'T FORGET, and archived it.

EPILOGUE

S O MUCH OF MY REFUGEE patients' health was influenced by external factors: housing, social connections, poverty, health insurance, employment, and access to trauma counselling. Most of this context in which patients live falls under the domain of public health, a field I became increasingly interested in during my time at the refugee clinic. I wanted to expand what I could do as a family physician, to move beyond retail medicine. I wanted to look at health through a wider lens and to work upstream to influence populations rather than individuals.

After a dozen years at Main and Broadway, the health authority moved the clinic across town, further east, to the city outskirts. It was far more accessible to patients, most of whom didn't live in Vancouver. It made my morning commute arduous. Everything shrank a little—the team, the exam rooms, parking options, morale. The move was layered onto the loss of clinic resources, years of advocating for adequate health insurance for refugees, and unending tales of trauma.

It was an opportunity to make some changes. I felt the nudge to redirect my career. A year after the Haddads left the clinic, so did I. I decided to pursue further medical training, and entered a residency in Public Health and Preventive Medicine at the University of British Columbia. I've maintained my family physician licence; I can't imagine anything replacing the satisfaction and privilege of the doctor-patient relationship. I want a public health practice that incorporates clinical care.

I still live in Deep Cove, although I have less time to putter in the yard and I don't run as often as I should. My son and three daughters still make me feel rich; so does Pete. My sleep has improved, but the worldwide refugee situation has not. I still think about my patients every day.

ACKNOWLEDGEMENTS

I AM DEEPLY GRATEFUL TO MY agent, Robert Mackwood, whom I had written off as out of my league before we were serendipitously connected. To my publisher, TouchWood Editions, and my editor, Lynne Van Luven. To my work family in Vancouver: physicians, nurses, counsellors, front desk staff, interpreters, settlement workers, and everyone else united by a commitment to do good hard work. To Pete and the kids—Saskia, Leif, Ariana, and Ilia—who were gracious enough to lower the volume when I had a sudden idea that needed to be dictated into my phone. And most of all, I am grateful to my patients, who taught me more than I bargained for. You brought me a lot of joy. I'm still looking out for you.

I'VE BEEN WRITING ABOUT MY clinical work—formally and informally—for years, and have been published in print and online. Some of those articles provided ideas or descriptions that were included or expanded upon in this book. I wish to thank *Mothers in Medicine* (mothersinmedicine .com), the *Canadian Medical Association Journal* (cmaj.ca), the College of Family Physicians of Canada's *Stories in Family Medicine* (http://www.cfpc.ca/Stories/), and the *San Francisco Medicine* journal (sfmms.org) for publishing earlier pieces. I'd also like to thank *Canadian Family Physician* (http://www.cfpc .ca/CanadianFamilyPhysician/) for publishing "The Birthday Party" in January 2017, and the *Province* (theprovince.com) for publishing my opinion piece "BC Needs to Improve Care for Refugees" on May 4, 2015.

NOTES

Chapter 1

[1] "Committee to Protect Journalists," https://www.cpj.org/killed/mideast/iraq/murder.php.

Chapter 2

[1] Mary Oliver, "Sometimes," in *Red Bird: Poems* (Boston: Beacon Press, 2008).

[2] Frederick Buechner, *Wishful Thinking: A Theological ABC* (New York: Harper & Row, 1973).

Chapter 3

[1] Melanie Tervalon, "Cultural Humility versus Cultural Competence: A Critical Distinction in Defining Physician Training Outcomes in Multicultural Education." *Journal of Health Care for the Poor and Underserved*, 9(2)(1998): 117–125.

[2] Wade Davis in Carol Black's *Schooling the World: The White Man's Last Burden*, documentary film, (Lost People Films, 2010), available at www. Schoolingtheworld.com.

Chapter 6

[1] Gabor Maté, *When the Body Says No: The Cost of Hidden Stress* (Canada: Vintage Canada, 2004).

[2] Mark E. Silverman, Jock T. Murray, & Charles S. Bryan, *The Quotable Osler* (American College of Physicians, 2002).

[3] William Wordsworth, "Nuns Fret Not at Their Convent's Narrow Room," in *The Sonnets of William Wordsworth* (London: Edward Moxon, 1838).

Chapter 7

[1] R. Edward Hendrick & Mark A. Helvie, "Mammography screening: A new estimate of number needed to screen to prevent one breast cancer death." *American Journal of Roentgenology*, 198(3) (March, 2012): 723–728, doi: 10.2214/AJR.11.7146.

[2] Kevin Pottie, Christina Greenaway, John Feightner et al, "Evidence-based Clinical Guidelines for Immigrants and Refugees." CMAJ (June, 2010): E1–E102, doi: 10.1503/cmaj.090313.

Chapter 8

[1] Phyllis Theroux, *California and other States of Grace* (New York: W. Morrow, 1980).

Chapter 11

[1] Cynthia Willard, Mara Rabin, & Martha Lawless, "The Prevalence of Torture and Associated Symptoms in United States Iraqi Refugees." *Journal of Immigrant and Minority Health*, 16(6) (December, 2014): 1069-76, doi: 10.1007/s10903-013-9817-5.

Chapter 14

[1] Michael Pollan, *Second Nature* (New York: Grove Press, 1991).
[2] "Mental Capital and Wellbeing: Making the Most of Ourselves in the 21st Century." (London: The Government Office for Science, 2008).

Chapter 15

[1] Susan Cain, *Quiet: The Power of Introverts in a World That Can't Stop Talking* (New York: Crown Publishers, 2012).

Chapter 17

[1] Jacqueline Thousand, Richard Villa, & Ann Nevin, *Creativity and Collaborative Learning: A Practical Guide to Empowering Students and Teachers* (Baltimore: Paul Brookes, 1994).

Chapter 24

[1] Christina August Hecht & Ernest B. Hook, "Rates of Down Syndrome at Livebirth by One-Year Maternal Age Intervals in Studies With Apparent Close to Complete Ascertainment in Populations of European Origin: A Proposed Revised Rate Schedule for Use in Genetic and Prenatal Screening." *American Journal of Medical Genetics*, 62(1996): 376-385.

Chapter 26

[1] Erik H. Erikson, *Childhood and Society* (New York: Norton, 1963).
[2] Henry David Thoreau, *Walden* (London: J.M. Dent, 1908).

Chapter 27

[1] "BC Needs to Improve Care for Refugees," the *Province*, May 4, 2015.

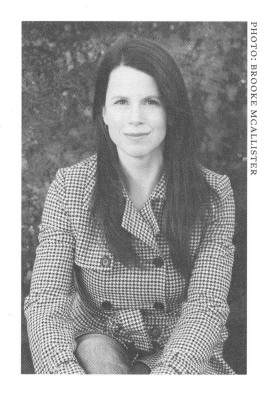

PHOTO: BROOKE MCALLISTER

DR. MARTINA SCHOLTENS is a clinical instructor with the Faculty of Medicine at the University of British Columbia and worked at the province's only refugee clinic for ten years, caring for patients from around the globe. The recipient of the Mimi Divinsky Award for History and Narrative in Family Medicine (2016), she is currently completing her Master of Public Health degree. Scholtens has done extensive advocacy work around federal health insurance for refugees, and has a special interest in narrative medicine. For more information, visit martinascholtens.com.